The Communion of the Holy Spirit

The Communion of the Holy Spirit

Watchman Nee
Translated from the Chinese

Christian Fellowship Publishers, Inc.
New York

ISBN: 978-0-935008-79-1

Available from the Publishers at:

11515 Allecingie Parkway
Richmond, Virginia 23235
www.c-f-p.com

Printed in the United States of America

Translator's Preface

The apostle Paul ends his second letter to the Corinthians with the divine salutation—"The grace of the Lord Jesus Christ, and the love of God, and the communion of the Holy Spirit, be with you all" (13.14). We as Christians come to know the fullness of the Godhead through the love, the grace and the communion which proceed from the triune God. It is the love of God the Father that purposes all. It is the grace of God the Son that provides all. And it is the communion of God the Spirit that performs all. Love, grace and communion are all equally essential. What would love be without grace? It would have no expression. What would grace be without communion? It would be unattainable.

This present volume is a compilation of messages given by God's servant Watchman Nee at various times and places. They all relate to the communion of the Holy Spirit. The first part consists of two messages on Resurrection, the Holy Spirit, and the Church. A proper perspective on the marvelous work of the Holy Spirit is therein given. The second part, entitled "The Outpouring of the Holy Spirit," is composed of six messages on the Outpouring, one message on the Holy Spirit, and the Law, and two messages on the Anointing Oil. And the third part presents four messages on Spiritual Judgment, which is the fruit of the discipline of the Holy Spirit. Such discipline gives spiritual discernment for service.

May the blessed Lord who released these messages to the Church use them for the building up of the body of Christ in love.

CONTENTS

Scripture quotations are from the
American Standard Version of the Bible
(1901), unless otherwise indicated.

PART ONE

RESURRECTION, THE HOLY SPIRIT, AND THE CHURCH*

* Part One consists of two messages that cover this multi-faceted subject. They were delivered in Chinese by the author at two successive Lord's Day gatherings of his fellow-workers on 13 June and 20 June 1948. These two gatherings, which met at the Conference Center on Mount Kuling just outside Foochow in southern China, were but two of many meetings that were held as part of the months-long First Workers Training Session which had its beginning in June and concluded in October of 1948. The contents of these two messages to follow have been derived from extensive notes taken down in Chinese by participants present at the Workers Conference, and have now been translated into English—Translator

PART ONE

RESURRECTION, THE HOLY SPIRIT, AND THE CHURCH

1: Resurrection, the Holy Spirit, and the Church (1)

In the Bible can be found three main subjects: resurrection, the Holy Spirit, and the Church. These three cannot be understood with the human mind because they are far beyond its comprehension. Nor can they be explained by human words. These three depend wholly on whatever the Spirit of the Lord gives us to see.

In order to know them we must begin with Genesis. We know that when man was created by the hand of God he was perfect and yet incomplete. All other created things were both perfect and complete. Man alone was perfect but not completed. The very fact that after God had created man He placed him before the tree of life and the tree of the knowledge of good and evil to let him choose between them proved that God's creation of man was still unfinished. In the eyes of God man was incomplete, for he could not yet distinguish between right and wrong. He still needed God's life as represented by the tree of life. Once man was made out of dust he still needed to add on God's life. Indeed, when man was created, he was living and yet he did not have God's life. This final step must be taken on by man himself. By taking in the life of God, as represented by the tree of life, he would then be completed. However, instead of eating of the tree of life, he ate of the tree of the knowledge of good and evil. Man had made the wrong choice, thus delaying the work of his completion.

For this reason, man did not attain to his highest level. In God's eyes, man was altogether wanting. Therefore, the entire Old Testament—from the first chapter of Genesis to the last chapter of Malachi—speaks of the extended work of God's creation. For however good Abraham, Isaac, Jacob, David and others might be, in the eyes of God they were all incomplete because they did not attain to His original plan of creation.

Though they had God's likeness, they did not have His image (likeness is outward appearance, whereas image is inward nature and character.)

Hence during the ensuing four thousand years God continues on with His work of the creation of man. At the same time God makes no further improvement on all his other created things. He has not thereafter created any superior flowers, birds, horses and other things, for these were created perfect and complete from the very beginning. On them there can be no more improvement, only man remains incomplete. In Genesis God is recorded as saying: "Let us make man in our image, after our likeness" (1.26a). Man was created in God's image and according to His likeness. "Likeness" refers to external form; it does not refer to internal quality. Adam, when created, became a living soul. He did not have God's Spirit in him. Hence, at this stage he was unfinished and incomplete. Adam was still in need of God himself to be his inward nature as was represented by the tree of life.

From the beginning of Genesis to the time of the Lord Jesus, no one had ever before attained to God's required standard of man. Adam looked like God in appearance, but he was not like God in character. The effect of his fall was to "fall short of the glory of God" (Rom. 3.23), thus forfeiting God's image. And so has it been with all who have followed Adam. Before the birth of our Lord Jesus there was not one typical or normal person in this world. No matter how the sages of the past disciplined and improved themselves, they failed to attain this goal. All fell short before God. It is by this, therefore, that we may understand the difference between the New and Old Testaments. The Old Testament shows that man has not attained to God's purpose, while the New Testament tells us that God's desired man is completed.

Thank God that the man whom He had longed for but had never before seen on earth is now seen and presented in the New Testament. That man, of course, is Christ. The one whom

God had sought out for so many years is now finally found in the person of the Lord Jesus. The Lord Jesus is the truly typical, normal man. He does not represent men but is himself the representative man. He is the Man whom God has always been after.

One—Resurrection

1. The need of resurrection.

When the Lord Jesus was on earth He was perfect in character but not absolute in power. Our Lord's power was restrained. Therefore, His thirty-three years of living on earth are incomplete unless He is resurrected. This is beyond our comprehension. Yet this is a tremendous event that requires revelation. Why must the Lord be raised from among the dead? Because during His days on earth He was restricted by time and space. For people to find Him they must go to His presence. They might even have to uncover the roof of a house to get to Him (see Mark 2.1-4). They had to press through the thronging multitude in order to merely touch His garment (see Mark 5.24-27). The Roman centurion was an exception. Of all men, he alone had an "unthronging" faith. The Lord commended it as "so great [a] faith": for he only asked for a word of healing from the Lord Jesus when his servant fell sick. And when the centurion professed his faith in acknowledging the Lord as being beyond the limitation of time and space, his servant got well instantly (see Luke 7.1-10). This centurion had revelation. Inasmuch as the Lord had been conceived and born of the Holy Spirit (see Matt. 1.20, Luke 1.35), He had in character reached the peak of God's created man. Even so, His power was restricted; and therefore, there is the need for resurrection.

13

2. In resurrection God obtains the representative man.

We now will see what resurrection is. Resurrection means that God has obtained the representative man: "Thou art my Son, this day have I begotten thee" (Heb.1.5). According to Acts 13.33-34, this same word is quoted within the context of speaking about the resurrection of the Lord Jesus. The meaning of resurrection is that Jesus the typical man is henceforth no longer subject to any limitation. He is to live forever. His resurrection transcends all natural restrictions. According to 1 Peter 1.3, we are born again "unto a living hope by the resurrection of Jesus Christ from the dead." While the Lord was on earth He had the possibility of death. After His resurrection, however, death is destroyed by Him. He now lives forever. Henceforth, the power of death as well as the possibility of death are both totally demolished.

Hallelujah! For four thousand years God had worked on man. But then, He finally got the man He longed for. God said to the Lord Jesus, "Thou art my Son, this day have I begotten thee" (see Heb. 1.1-5, Acts 13.33-34, Ps. 2.7). God declared this at the resurrection of the Lord Jesus. When the Lord was born in Bethlehem, God had not said this. It was only when He was raised from among the dead that God joyfully declared, "Thou art my Son, this day have I begotten thee." Hence, we see that at the Lord's resurrection God finally possesses the Man of His heart.

3. Resurrection eliminated the restriction of time and space.

What is resurrection? Resurrection is the breaking through by a person of all restrictions, even breaking through the strongest restriction which is death. In resurrection Jesus breaks through all barriers. The New Testament mentions the dead being raised a number of times—such as in the instance of the only son of the woman in Nain (Luke 7.11-15); the little daughter of Jairus, a ruler of the synagogue (Matt. 9.18-25, cf.

Mark 5.22ff.), and Lazarus (John 11). Yet even in the case of Lazarus, it is only resuscitation or the returning of the soul. He was still bound with grave clothes that needed to be loosened before he could walk. And Lazarus, like the others, eventually had to die. Only the resurrection of the Lord Jesus is of a kind that is not bound by death. He is risen and dies no more. In the record of the whole Bible, only the Lord is resurrected.

When brother T. Austin-Sparks of England spoke of the Lord's resurrection, he once said this: that with respect to the resurrected Lord, there is neither come nor go; for no one sees from where He comes nor knows to where He goes; He merely appears and disappears at various times; and hence, He does not come, He appears; He does not go, He disappears. The problem lies not in His coming and going, but rather depends instead on our seeing or not seeing Him. In the record of John 20 we are told that at the early morn of His resurrection the Lord Jesus said to Mary Magdalene, "Touch me not" (vv.16-17). This is because He is now different from the past. When He told Thomas to touch His side this became for him a matter of faith. Jesus wanted Thomas to touch Him with faith. Touching the resurrected Lord by faith makes Him touchable. As regards the risen Lord, apart from revelation there is no question of coming or going. The greatest restrictions of man are those of time and space. Yet neither of these can limit the Lord. Resurrection has transcended all restrictions. Hallelujah, today our Lord Jesus is absolutely unlimited. If we live in the Holy Spirit, we can touch the Lord. The Lord is in our midst. All obstructions have been eliminated.

It was after Lazarus had breathed his last breath that the Lord Jesus began His travel back into Judea from the other side of the river Jordan. When He finally arrived at the home of Lazarus, Martha said to Him, "Lord, if thou hadst been here, my brother had not died." The Lord answered, "Thy brother shall rise again." Her response was, "I know that he shall rise again in the resurrection at the last day." The Lord Jesus immediately replied, "I am the resurrection, and the life: he that believeth on me, though he die, yet shall he live ... Believest thou this?" (John 11.1-26) What the Lord meant here is: "I am the last day! If you believe, you shall see resurrection now. Where I am, time does not exist, neither is there the last day." Concerning resurrection, there is not the factor of time. Outside of resurrection, time is a big problem. But with resurrection, time is no longer an issue because it is not circumscribed by time.

Not only this, resurrection is also unrestricted by space. We remember how the two disciples on the road to Emmaus saw the risen Lord. Meanwhile, the other disciples back in Jerusalem also saw the resurrected Lord (see Luke 24.13-35). The Son of God has resurrected; He has transcended geography and time. So with respect to Him after His resurrection, there is no before or after time. He is not bound by any timetable. To Him nothing ever occurs three or five years later. The issues of time and space no longer exist. Today people throughout the entire earth may touch Him at the   same time.

4. The power of resurrection is the supreme power.

The greatest restriction on earth is death. There is nothing that is not under its control. Death is the limitation to all living beings. But in His resurrection, the Lord Jesus destroys the restriction of death. Though death is the greatest limitation, resurrection overcomes it. Resurrection, therefore, is the greatest power. If we touch the power of resurrection, we can easily cover all of China with the gospel of the kingdom.

Two—the Holy Spirit

1. Transmit the resurrected Lord.

What about the Holy Spirit? When Peter preached the gospel to the Jews, he said: "Being therefore by the right hand of God exalted, and having received of the Father the promise of the Holy Spirit, he [Christ Jesus] hath poured forth this, which ye see and hear" (Acts 2.33). Resurrection places the Lord at the right hand of God; and while He sits at the Father's right hand, He pours forth the Holy Spirit. Thus, the power of the Holy Spirit is also the power of resurrection. This is to say that in the Holy Spirit the Lord pours forth resurrection together with the power of His resurrection. Hence, whoever touches the Spirit touches resurrection. As soon as a person is in the Holy Spirit he touches the resurrected Lord. The Holy Spirit testifies to the resurrection of the Lord.

When our Lord was on earth some leaned upon His breast, some kissed Him, some thronged Him, some received things from His hand. He washed people's feet and touched their hands. During that time, though people were able to touch the Lord, their touch was far inferior to our touch today. For we are no longer restricted by time and space. Today, the risen Lord is in the Holy Spirit. What we thus see today far surpasses what they saw before. The Church is able to continue on for two thousand years due to the seeing of the Lord clearly within men. What we see outwardly may not be as clear as what those saw in the time of the record of the Gospels; yet inwardly our knowledge of the Lord exceeds that of that earlier time. The moment we are in the Spirit we immediately touch the Lord.

The prime work of the Holy Spirit is to transmit the resurrected Lord to us. He does not convey the Christ as recorded in the Gospels; He transmits the resurrected Christ. When people met the Lord while He was on earth they could only say how tall was His stature, how wise He was, and how old He looked. Some could say at one point in the Lord's earthly life that He was only twelve years old or that they had seen His brothers in the flesh. But now in the Holy Spirit we are no longer restricted by time and space, and what we touch is also the Christ who is beyond time and space.

17

2. The power of resurrection is in the Holy Spirit.

The Lord transcends all restrictions. The Holy Spirit today comes to testify to the transcendent Christ. If someone declares that he knows the Holy Spirit and yet today he does not know the resurrected Christ who transcends all, he is one who has not known the Christ in the Holy Spirit. For the power of resurrection is in the Holy Spirit. Ephesians 1.21 declares that the resurrected Christ is "far above all rule, and authority, and power, and dominion, and every name that is named, not only in this world, but also in that which is to come." God has made the risen Lord to sit at His right hand and caused Him to transcend everything known and unknown to men. All that can be named has been surpassed by the Lord, not only in this world but also in that world to come. Resurrection breaks through all barriers. Normally only the everlasting transcends all. But God plans to allow the mortal to transcend also. The work of the Holy Spirit today is to reveal this resurrection power in us. We should recognize that the Holy Spirit is the Spirit of resurrection. The Spirit who transcends all is the Holy Spirit.

Three—the Church

1. Resurrection power moves and is stored up in the Church.

Let us speak of the Church. What is it? The Church means that the Lord is the Head and we are the Body. What, then, is the relationship between the Church and resurrection? What is the Church's relationship with the Holy Spirit? Ephesians 1.19-20 speaks of the exceeding greatness of the power which God wrought in Christ when He raised the Lord Jesus from the dead. Yet the Church is where this same power also works. Let us take note of the word "according" in verse 19: "what the exceeding greatness of his power to us-ward who believe, according to that working of the strength of his might which he wrought in Christ." In other words, the exceeding greatness of God's power which works in Christ works also in us the Church. The mighty power which the Church is now experiencing is the same as Christ had experienced. The Church and Christ are not only the same in nature, they are the same in power. Otherwise, the Church is empty. The way by which God broke through all limitations in the Lord is the same way God will enable the Church to break through all barriers.

Therefore, the Church today should have the same power and enjoy the same liberty, uninhibited by anything, just as the risen Lord himself had. Otherwise, it cannot be considered the Church. The exceedingly great power of God works not just in Christ, it continues to work today also in the Church. The Church is the reservoir of the power of resurrection today. This is the Church. Nothing less is acceptable. The Church is the body of Christ; accordingly it should not fall short of this exceedingly great power.

This is followed by Ephesians 1.22-23 which states that God had not only raised Christ from the dead and made Him far above all, but also that God "put all things in subjection under his feet, and gave him to be head over all things to the church." Jesus is risen and glorified. He is no longer the humble Nazarene. He is the victorious Christ. All things today are subject to Him. While He was on earth He was the perfect man. He was Head, but not yet the glorified Head; for at that time the possibility of death had yet to be broken. Many Bible teachers try to find the Church in the four Gospels. But the Church cannot be found in the Gospels (see below) because the account therein is of a Jesus who was still restricted. Had the Church been related only to the earthly life of Jesus, she would be merely a limited institution. We think it is enough to possess the Lord's earthly power and authority, but God pronounces this to be insufficient. God led Christ through death and resurrection, and then through the coming of the Holy Spirit deposited that resurrection power in the Church.

Today the Church receives its supply of power in the ascended and glorified Christ. Therefore, there is no problem the Church cannot solve and no temptation the Church cannot overcome. For the power of the Church is the power of the resurrection of Christ—that which subdues all things under His feet. Her power is no less than the power which had been wrought in Christ.

When Christ was on earth, there was no Church. For then He had not been resurrected and everything was yet under restriction. After Christ was raised from the dead, had ascended up to heaven and poured out the Holy Spirit, the Church was born. The Lord is risen, so the Church becomes the body of Christ, being filled with the nature, and becoming the vessel, of the resurrected Christ. Christ is the Head, and the Church as His body is the fullness of Him who fills all in all. As Christ is, so is the Church. As Christ is unrestricted, so the Church is not restricted. There is no better analogy to describe Christ and the Church than that of the human body. In the latter, the head and all its members share one life, having one nature. And to be the body, all its members must be present. So is it with the body of Christ. I may make a chair short of one leg, but the body of Christ cannot be short of any leg, arm or whatever.

2. The Holy Spirit manifests
the resurrection power of Christ in the Church.

We believers are made to drink of one Holy Spirit. The same Spirit causes us to be the body of Christ. For this reason, wherever two persons on earth touch the resurrection of Christ, what they bind shall be bound and what they loose shall be loosed (see Matt. 18.18-20). The minimum of the Church is two persons. If, then, two can touch the power of resurrection and stand on the ground of resurrection, they can command all situations. In former days the Church was ignorant of this potential, hence it probably took decades to make any progress. Now that we know what the Church is, we can make great strides. Even your personal, impossible situation will be quickly resolved. For the Church is the reservoir of the power of the resurrection of Christ.

What is the work of the Holy Spirit today? The Spirit today is manifesting the resurrection power of Christ in the Church. All problems are now solved: "the gates of Hades shall not prevail against" the Church, said the Lord (Matt. 18.18b). I personally am persuaded that this word suggests that all the gates of Hades shall be open towards the Church; and yet these gates shall not prevail against the Church. Why? Because Hades represents death, whereas the Church represents resurrection. The Church shall therefore prevail.

Hence, for the Lord to have His way on earth today, it lies not in how much our walk has changed, or in how much truth we know, but in whether there are people who really are willing to pay any cost to know resurrection, the Holy Spirit, and the Church. But if so, the Church shall have a glorious testimony.

In Practice

In practice each one of us has already experienced something of resurrection, since the salvation of any soul is the work of resurrection. On the other hand, people may endure suffering, and even die a martyr's death, for the Lord. All of this is because of the power of resurrection. First Corinthians 15 is a chapter in the Scriptures on the truth of resurrection. It concludes with the word, "always abounding in the work of the Lord" (v.58b), which work is done in the power of resurrection. It is also in this power of resurrection that people bear the cross, receive spiritual edification, see some light, and arrive   at holiness.

During the last two thousand years these truths have been brought—here a little, there a little—to today's understanding. If today people would stand on this resurrection ground, there would be a great result. I have an idea that people today do not see sufficiently enough of the Lord's resurrection.

The Lord is powerful. He transcends all things and is able to break down every barrier. Yet He is but the Head. What is marvelous is that today God wants us to be joined with the Lord in one. Such a New Man in Christ is beyond restriction and is well able to manifest the power of God. Oh, this is such a tremendous thing. Unless in our day we have this revelation we will not be able to make any advance in testimony. Were we to receive some light before the Lord so as to see, we would save much time and energy. May the Lord be merciful to us and open our eyes that we may see resurrection, the Holy Spirit, and the Church and their interrelatedness.

2: Resurrection, the Holy Spirit, and the Church (2)

Death Is the Greatest Restriction

Last Lord's Day we spoke on Resurrection, the Holy Spirit, and the Church. Today we want to speak further about these matters. What we saw last Lord's Day was that death is the greatest restriction. We want to reinforce this word. All living creatures end at death. Accordingly, for all living things the ultimate limitation is death. Small animals end at death, but so do the big animals. All living things, from plants to animals, are altogether circumscribed by death. Yet this is also true with respect to human beings. Man's intellect may advance considerably, such as in the case of the rich man spoken of in one of the parables of the Lord Jesus (in it, interestingly enough, God addressed the rich man as, "Thou foolish one"). The advanced intellect of this rich man enables him to plan and plot for his future, but he is finished and done for when God requires his soul (see Luke 12.16-21). Many of our loved ones—such as our fathers, mothers and children—have died. And once having died, they are never recalled to life. But so many great men suffered the same consequence; however powerful and influential they were in their lives, they too died and are gone. Hence, death is the greatest restriction.

Resurrected Man Is God's Appointed Man

When the Lord Jesus was on earth He was the representative man. During His forty days after resurrection He was still the representative man. In His thirty-three years on earth He was the representation of morality, but in His first forty days after resurrection He stood as the representation of power. In fact, these forty days manifested His power. Fundamental theologians view the Lord Jesus on earth as the typical or standard man. They correctly deduce that if the Lord had not died for us God would for sure have condemned us for our sins because we have all fallen below the standard, and are thus under condemnation. Had Christ not died and the veil in the temple not been rent, God would have condemned us for our sins instead of having saved us. But past theologians did not clearly see the truth surrounding the resurrection of Christ. Only in this century have people begun to see resurrection truth in a fuller light. Resurrected man alone is God's man of design: "Thou art my Son, this day have I begotten thee" (Heb. 1.5). As we have indicated already, this declaration by God has reference to the time when the Lord Jesus was risen and came out of the tomb. After the Lord was resurrected and had emerged from the tomb, God said to Him, "This day have I begotten thee." It was there and then that God obtained the Man of His heart desire.

Our being the children of God also begins with the resurrection of Christ. Ever since the fall of man we human beings have all come short of the glory of God (see Rom. 3.23). Except for resurrection, we cannot be saved. Of all human beings the Lord Jesus alone has not fallen short of God's glory for He is the perfect man. However, besides His desire for a perfect man God had an added desire that this perfect man must be a man of power. God wants a powerful man as well as a moral man. From the moment of His birth on earth in Bethlehem, the Lord is a man of morality. But from the moment of His resurrection He has manifested himself as a man of power; for after His resurrection Christ is able to be omnipresent. Time and space can no longer limit Him since He has become a man with resurrection power. Thus does the Lord Jesus fulfill God's plan in the creation of man and becomes the Man of God's desire.

Resurrection Transcends All

After His resurrection, the Lord is not only unrestricted by time and space but is also unbound by death. He has broken the barrier of death. The rising of Lazarus from the dead is different from the Lord's resurrection: with Lazarus it is but a resuscitation, not a real resurrection: he was still bound by grave clothes and eventually he died: the power of death was yet upon him. At the resurrection of the Lord, however, the boundary of death was broken through by Him, "because it was not possible that he should be holden of it [held in its power]" (Acts 2.24). The gates of Hades could not close against Him nor swallow Him up. Christ is risen and He dies no more. Death has no power upon Him.

When the Lord was resurrected, even His disciples, such as Peter and Thomas, did not believe it. Mary Magdalene ran and reported to Peter and John that the Lord was not to be found in the tomb. These two immediately left to investigate. They saw "the linen cloths lying, and the napkin, that was upon his head, not lying with the linen cloths, but rolled up in a place by itself"; yet the Lord was not there (see John 20.1-8). In the case of Lazarus coming out of the tomb, we know that he was still "bound hand and foot with grave-clothes" and "his face was bound about with a napkin"; he was still under limitation (see John 11.44). But at the Lord's resurrection, the linen grave clothes and napkin were left in the tomb, yet He himself had departed. This indicates that the Lord has transcended all restrictions. And hence His resurrection is essentially different from that of Lazarus.

Brother Sparks had two words about the Lord and resurrection: It is not His coming but His appearing; it is not His going, but His disappearing. Since His resurrection, nothing can confine Him. In Christ Jesus nothing can limit Him, neither death, nor time, nor space, nor anything else. Not only that, after He was resurrected, the Lord Jesus was exalted by God to the highest place, seated in heaven at the Father's right hand, "far above all rule, and authority, and power, and dominion, and every name that is named, not only in this world, but also in that which is to come" (Eph. 1.20-21). Consequently, the resurrected Christ transcends all. Today the Lord is leading us, on the one hand, to be as moral as He is and, on the other hand, to have resurrection power such as He has. The man whom God desires is morally, as well as powerfully, perfect.

The Church: Born of the Spirit after the Lord's Resurrection to Be the Body of the Resurrected Christ, Joined in One with the Head

It is after His resurrection that Christ became the Head of the Church. Before His resurrection, He was on earth as a man; He had not become the Head of the Church. Only after resurrection did He ascend up to the Father and receive the promised Holy Spirit, whom He then poured forth to give birth to the Church. The Lord is resurrected in order to be the Head of the Church as well as to join us believers together to be the Body. God now makes Christ the Head and us the body of Christ. Just as the nature of the human head is, so is the nature of the human body. The word of God shows us that just as the Lord is in resurrection so the Church is in resurrection. Hence what is the Church? It is that which holds the resurrection of Christ.

The Church is built on resurrection ground, or else it cannot be reckoned as the Church. Ephesians 1.19-20a speaks of "the exceeding greatness of his [God's] power to us-ward who believe, according to that working of the strength of his might which he wrought in Christ, when he raised him from the dead." Today this same resurrection power works in us. This power in Christ makes Him the Head; this same power in us makes us the Body. This is what the Church is. Hence, unless we experience the power of the resurrection of Christ we do not know what the Church is. The Church should not be restricted at all, but should overcome everything just as Christ has.

Why is it that the letter to the Ephesians is considered to be the book in the Bible which uncovers the height of truth? Because it reveals the body of Christ. In nature and in power the body of Christ is the same as Christ. Yet to understand the body of Christ we need revelation. Otherwise, what we profess to know about the Church is but a matter of terminology. We need to stand on the ground of the Church experientially. There should be at least two persons who together touch that resurrection power of Christ and pray with one accord. The word of the Lord is clear: "All authority hath been given unto me in heaven and on earth" (Matt. 28.19-20). Today the Lord entrusts us with the execution of this authority. This is because we are His body. Besides the fact of our still being in these earthly mortal bodies, there is also the fact that we are joined to the Lord in one spirit. We are not different from the Lord spiritually. What a tremendous reality this is!

Need the Spirit of Wisdom and Revelation

When we see what resurrection is, we become clear about what the Body is. After His resurrection the Lord poured forth the Holy Spirit to give birth to the Church. He becomes the Head, and the Church becomes His body. How all-important is the Body! There is nothing higher than that a person would be willing to accept others to be members of his body. Just so, the Lord Jesus accepts us to be members of His body and He gives us His authority to exercise. How great is the Lord!

Brother Sparks also said this: the work of the Holy Spirit is found wherever the resurrection power of the Lord is working; otherwise, it cannot be reckoned as His work. Once again, it must be said that this cannot be comprehended by the human mind. We must pray and ask God to grant us the spirit of wisdom and revelation. What we need today is this revelation, the revelation concerning the power which God has already given us. If there be two or three believers with this revelation and praying with one accord on the ground of resurrection, they can execute the authority of heaven.

Hallelujah, today we do not need to have more of what we already have; rather, we need to see how glorious, rich and great that indeed is which we already have. Heavenly authority is glorious and exceedingly great, but it is being restricted by earth. If today, however, two persons on earth recognize resurrection and stand on resurrection ground, they can shake the ends of the earth. Now we are merely touching the hem of the resurrection garment, for only in these recent years have we begun to have the word of the Lord on resurrection. Praise God! What He has revealed to us uncovers the height of Biblical truth: that we are one with the Lord! The problem today is on our side. May we all humble ourselves before God and pray: "O God, grant us the spirit of wisdom and revelation so that we may see."

PART TWO

THE OUTPOURING OF THE HOLY SPIRIT*

---

* The nine messages which comprise this Part were delivered in Chinese by the author at either Chuenchow or Shanghai in China between 1935 and 1942, as will be more specifically indicated at the beginning of each message. The contents of these nine messages to follow have been derived from extensive notes taken down in Chinese by those who were present at the meetings concerned, and have now been translated into English.— Translator

1: Outpouring of the Holy Spirit Explained*

Concerning the outpouring of the Holy Spirit, it is a subject that is not easy to explain. Being limited in time, we can only share a little today. This, however, does not mean that the Bible has only this much on the subject. We can only scan through the material; we cannot conduct an in-depth study. Nevertheless, let us study as much as we can on the one hand and pray much on the other. May God give us more light.

Outpouring of Holy Spirit
vs. Outpouring of Evil Spirit

With regard to the outward appearance of the outpouring of the Holy Spirit, many wonder about some "abnormal" or unusual phenomena. In the Bible, such phenomena are truly mentioned. Over the past eight or nine years as I have studied this subject, I discovered that these manifestations are indeed in the Bible. Nevertheless, abnormal or unusual phenomena in and of themselves do not necessarily prove the genuineness of the outpouring of the Holy Spirit. The biblical proof is found in 1 Corinthians 12.1-3. Verse 1 speaks of spiritual gifts. However, we find that the English word "gifts" has been placed in italics in the text, which indicates that this word is not in the original Greek. So Paul is not speaking here of spiritual gifts. The Greek word pneumatikos here is equivalent to "spiritualities" or "spiritual inspirations." Govett, Pember, Panton, and other Biblical scholars translate this as "being inspired"; that is to say, the spirit in question comes upon a person, thus causing strange movement or manifestation. In verse 2, "led away" originally refers to a being inspired by the evil spirit. And hence, in the

---

* Notes of message given at Chuenchow, Fukien Province 18 November 1935.—Translator

original this phrase does not point to a being led away according to the common, ordinary understanding; rather, it has to do with supernatural matters. Paul wants the Corinthian believers to know about spiritual inspiration.

In our brief study today we shall come to see the difference between the outpouring of the Holy Spirit and the outpouring of the evil spirit. Paul has not told us here of the outward manifestations of these two outpourings. He certainly knows, but he does not explain. In spite of his omission, though, we still need to pay attention to them. Outwardly these two outpourings are quite difficult to distinguish, yet inwardly the differences are great.

The Two Outpourings Differ in Speech

The main difference between the outpouring of the Holy Spirit and that of the evil spirit lies in the area of speech, not in body movement, attitude and so forth: "No man speaking in the Spirit of God saith, Jesus is anathema; and no man can say, Jesus is Lord, but in the Holy Spirit" (1 Cor. 12.3). Whether or not a person receives the outpouring of the Holy Spirit can be recognized by the word of his mouth. Only those who are inspired by the Holy Spirit can say that Jesus is Lord. This cannot be falsified. Unless a person is inspired by the Holy Spirit, he is not able to say "Jesus is Lord." He who cannot say this is definitely being poured upon by the evil spirit. When a spirit comes upon a person, we can use this method to examine and test that spirit. He who can say "Jesus is Lord" has the outpouring of the Holy Spirit. On the other hand, he who cannot say "Jesus is Lord" is poured upon by the evil spirit. If when a person is challenged, and he moves away, it becomes doubtful that he has been poured upon by the Holy Spirit. But if he can say, "Lord, I am unworthy, this is Your grace," he is being inspired by the Holy Spirit.

Yet do not doubt simply because there are sometimes "abnormalities." If inspiration is common and regular, it is no more inspiration. He who is inspired by the Holy Spirit has the Spirit upon him. Hence he should be somewhat different from the ordinary.

Holy Spirit and Evil Spirit
Differ in Working Principle

We may also judge the difference between the outpouring of the Holy Spirit and that of the evil spirit by the diverse working principles involved. In order for the evil spirit to be poured out upon a person two conditions are required. First, there must be a passive will. One with a passive will can easily give ground to an evil spirit. For this reason, Christians should not be passive. Second, there must be a vacant mind. The minds of many are idle. These people are unwilling to exercise their own minds. Such people can also be easily deceived by evil spirits. So then, the outpouring of the Holy Spirit differs profoundly in principle from that of an evil spirit. The main differences are in the stances taken by the human will and mind. People who receive the outpouring of the Holy Spirit have these two characteristics: first, their minds are clear; second, their wills are not passive. They themselves are active, not allowing outside forces to work upon them. The Holy Spirit always requests a believer to actively exercise his will to cooperate with Him. How distinctly different is His working from that of the evil spirit who requires man's will to be passive. Thus can we judge whether it is the outpouring of the Holy Spirit or the outpouring of the evil spirit.

Conditions for Seeking the Spirit's Outpouring

1. Without hidden or undealt sins.

For us to seek for the outpouring of the Holy Spirit, there are certain conditions we must fulfill. First of all, we must not have any hidden or undealt sin before the Lord. If a person seeking the outpouring of the Holy Spirit has hidden sin in him, he is open to be deceived by evil spirits. This is because he gives ground in his heart to the evil spirit.

2. With an active will.

Secondly, for the Holy Spirit to come upon us, He requires the active desire of our will. Only then will He come. Not so with the evil spirit, who does not need our active desire but will come when the will is passive. Some people may pray, "If this is the Holy Spirit, this I claim. If it is the evil spirit, this I reject." Such prayer is still not positive enough with regard to the Holy Spirit. Our cooperation with the Spirit is like this: When the Holy Spirit comes upon you, He will probably ask you with a still, small voice within you, how much you will allow Him to come. In the measure of your allowance will be the measure of His coming. The power of decision is with you. Whatever is contrary to this is being passive, and is therefore not the work of the Holy Spirit but the work of the evil spirit. For the Holy Spirit to come upon you, you yourself must express your desire, and so He comes. It is not the Holy Spirit working independently. It is you who works actively and the Spirit comes to help. The Holy Spirit makes me laugh because I have begun to laugh. He then gives me power to laugh. This is what I mean by cooperation. As you seek the outpouring of the Spirit, you need to ask the Lord to cover you with His precious blood. You do your part, and the Spirit will most definitely do His part.

There was a brother who held himself tightly. He prayed, "Holy Spirit, if You want to come, come." After having prayed for several hours, the Spirit had not yet come upon him. Such prayer of his did not fulfill the working condition of the Holy Spirit; and thus, He did not come upon him. For the Spirit to work, He demands the cooperation of our will; otherwise, He will not work. This is like horse riding. The bridle of the horse is in the hand of the rider. When the bridle is loosened, the horse leaps forward. Nevertheless, the bridle is still in the rider's hand. This same principle works with respect to the outpouring of the Holy Spirit. On the one hand, we must let loose and give liberty to Him; on the other hand, we still need to cooperate with our will, or else we will lose all control.

Why the Holy Spirit Is Poured Forth

We also need to know why we must have the outpouring of the Holy Spirit. Peter, speaking to an assembly of Jews in Jerusalem, said, as recorded in Acts 2.33: "Being therefore by the right hand of God exalted, and having received of the Father the promise of the Holy Spirit, he [the risen and ascended Lord] hath poured forth this, which ye see and hear." And in verse 36 Peter continued by saying: "Let all the house of Israel therefore know assuredly, that God hath made him both Lord and Christ, this Jesus whom ye crucified." The "therefore" in verse 36 connects directly to verse 33 which tells of the exaltation of our Lord. Because of the Lord's exaltation the Holy Spirit was poured forth, just as what those Jews who listened to Peter both saw and heard on that Pentecost Day. In other words, the house of Israel ought to know that the outpouring of the Holy Spirit is the evidence of the exaltation and victory of Jesus the Nazarene. Had the Lord not been highly exalted, the Spirit would not possibly have been poured forth. Now that God has anointed Jesus of Nazareth and set Him as Lord and Christ, there is no possibility of not having the outpouring of the Holy Spirit. We receive the Spirit's outpouring, not to prove our faith and victory, but to prove that Jesus is Lord and Christ.

35

Praise and thank the Lord! Since His exaltation is a fact, the outpouring of the Holy Spirit is also a fact. Conversely, if the Lord has not been exalted, the Holy Spirit will not be able to be poured forth. Our Lord had been crucified and had shed His precious blood for the remission of sins. Therefore, all who believe in Him shall have their sins forgiven. By the same token, though, how can we say that He has been exalted to be Lord and Christ and yet we do not have the outpouring of the Holy Spirit? This is impossible! So then, let us boldly assert that the Lord has been exalted to the throne, and therefore, let Him fill us. We need to draw near in fullness of faith, believing in the Lord and what He has accomplished.

2: Conditions for the Spirit's Outpouring— and Important Matters to Watch[*]

As we have said before, in order to receive the outpouring of the Holy Spirit certain conditions must be fulfilled. First, there should be no conscious undealt sin in the heart; second, there must be hunger in the spirit: "I will pour water upon him that is thirsty, and streams upon the dry ground; I will pour my Spirit upon thy seed, and my blessing upon thine offspring" (Is. 44.3); and third, there needs to be fervent prayers: "These all with one accord continued steadfastly in prayer" (Acts 1.14a); "when the day of Pentecost was now come, they were all together in one place.

And they were all filled with the Holy Spirit . . ." (Acts 2.1,4); "they, when they heard it, lifted up their voice to God with one accord . . . And when they had prayed, the place was shaken wherein they were gathered together; and they were all filled with the Holy Spirit . . ." (Acts 4.24,31); "when the apostles that were at Jerusalem heard that Samaria had received the word of God, they sent unto them Peter and John: who, when they were come down, prayed for them, that they might receive the Holy Spirit: for as yet it was fallen upon none of them: only they had been baptized into the name of the Lord Jesus. Then laid they their hands on them, and they received the Holy Spirit" (Acts 8.14-17).

Matters to Be Watched on Receiving the Outpouring

In receiving the outpouring of the Holy Spirit, a person is brought into contact with things in the spiritual realm. Formerly things in the spiritual realm were rather vague and abstract to

[*] Notes of message given at Chuenchow, Fukien Province, again on 18 November 1935.—Translator

him. Now, though, with the outpouring of the Holy Spirit, one begins to be opened up to the spiritual realm, and hence he commences to contact things in that realm. Some may have faith, but they are unwilling to open the door. Their resistance keeps them from touching things in the spiritual realm. Seeking the outpouring of the Holy Spirit is like opening the door along a wall. After such opening there will be constant contact with things within the spiritual realm. This is viewing the matter from the good side. But viewing it from the bad side, there is also danger in being exposed to the spiritual realm. It can be likened to opening the door for friends to come in; but in the meanwhile, robbers may also slip in. Yet do not consider closing the door forever simply because robbers may get in. No, on the one hand, you must open the door; but on the other hand, you must be watchful.

Test the Spirits

How do you watch and not allow the wicked ones who inhabit the spiritual realm to enter in? First of all, each time you experience the outpouring of the Holy Spirit you must apply the test. You should not be negligent in this matter. In 1 Corinthians 12.3 and 1 John 4.3 the way of testing is mentioned. This is your security. You must challenge the person being poured upon by asking if Christ has come in the flesh. Or by asking him if Jesus is Lord. Watch to see if he withdraws. If so, it must be an evil spirit. If he can say that Jesus is Lord, then it is of the Holy Spirit. You should not test this out only nine out of ten times: you must test it out every time. On this matter, I think I have done my duty. Now you need to walk before God in this straight path.

According to the Principles of 1 Corinthians 14

The manifestation of the outpouring of the Holy Spirit is often exceptional on the first occasion. It seems as though God is being lenient with you so as to let you gain more. The first experience can be likened to passing through a gateway that leads to a house. After the gateway has been crossed, your life at home becomes quiet and tranquil. You have no need to leap or to be noisy, nor do you need to seek again for strange sensation and experience. Henceforth, you do not follow the principle in Acts 2; rather, you will follow the principles laid down in 1 Corinthians 14. We read there that in the assembly of the church the outpouring of the Holy Spirit is for building up others, not for self-building. Moreover, the spirits of the prophets are subject to the prophets (v.32). We need to learn to control our spirits. "If any man speaketh in a tongue, let it be by two, or at the most three, and that in turn" (v.27). We see from Acts 2 that the hundred and twenty speak simultaneously; for this was the first time. Henceforth, however, the principles set forth in 1 Corinthians 14 must be followed.

Control the Spirit

Whom you and I must obey is the indwelling Holy Spirit, for the indwelling Spirit is a Person; and since He has personality, we must yield ourselves to Him. But the spirit that is outpoured upon us is without personality and is therefore subject to us (see again 1 Cor. 14.32): we can allow it or not allow it to stay and we can also regulate its measure. Yet because the spirit that falls upon us is without personality, being instead a kind of manifestation, we must be careful to maintain control of the situation; for if we are not watchful, Satan may bring in a counterfeit. Indeed, because some believers have carelessly given the spirit that was upon them the control over them, confusing phenomena have resulted.

Let us be fully aware that though we obey the Spirit who dwells in us we ourselves govern the spirit that falls upon us. When we seek the outpouring of the Holy Spirit, whether that be at home or in the assembly, we must control that which is poured out upon us.

Exercise after Receiving the Outpouring

As to the exercise a person should engage in after experiencing the outpouring of the Holy Spirit, there are two facets to consider.[*] The first facet to consider is that it is best for you to use this power immediately by helping Christians and sinners. Formerly, you had no power to preach the gospel or edify believers. Today, though, you must use this newly-received power to preach the gospel and edify the saints. If you do not use this power, you will be like the evil servant who buried his one talent in the ground. No, upon receiving this power of the Holy Spirit, go and preach the gospel, and be an overcomer of the gospel. The reason why believers suffer failure in this area is because some among them treat the experience of the outpouring of the Holy Spirit as amusement. They seek the Spirit's outpouring merely to speak in tongues or to have a hearty laugh and then go home without applying the power possessed. The outpouring of the Holy Spirit is not for our amusement, but is an aid given to us to live and work for the Lord.

---

[*] It needs to be noted that to those who have not experienced the victorious life, this outpouring of the Holy Spirit will have little effect on their walk: it will fade away after but a few days. Such a situation can be likened to a tire that leaks air, soon making the bicycle immovable. Such is the condition of those without the experience of a victorious life but who receive the outpouring of the Holy Spirit for the first time. And if such be your experience, you should ask the Spirit to be outpoured once more. Whenever you feel cold, you need to seek the outpouring again.—Author

The other facet to consider is that the outpouring of the Holy Spirit is the best time for us to ask God for gifts. That is the time when we should ask God for the grace and gifts we need. Indeed, it is permissible for us to be more covetous in asking. Yet we must not boast about the experience we have had of the outpouring of the Holy Spirit. We should not brag before men; instead, let the grace and power of God be manifested so that He may be glorified more.

Giving Testimony Once Receiving the Outpouring

A few things must be noted about giving testimony to the outpouring of the Holy Spirit. First of all, when someone asks you about your experience of the outpouring, you should not disclose the details of your experience. When you give testimony, you should relate your testimony according to the following rules:

(1) Do not share the details. The book of Acts records the stories of many who had received the outpouring of the Holy Spirit. There were varied manifestations, such as speaking in tongues, preaching the gospel with great power, etc. But nowhere does it tell us these experiences in detail. Apart from several descriptions of the external evidences of the Spirit's outpouring, there is no mentioning of the detailed contents. Confusion is caused by accompanying the stories of the outpouring of the Holy Spirit with details.

(2) Do not overemphasize your experience. Those who long to know about the outpouring of the Holy Spirit are often very curious. They will not be helped by listening to stories of the outpouring. On the other hand, if you tell your own experience, it is easy for you to make your own experience the standard. In fact, however, the manifestation of the outpouring of the Holy Spirit varies from person to person. You must therefore not overstress your own experience.

(3) Another point to be made here is that in this matter of seeking for the Spirit's outpouring some groups of believers emphasize "ask" whereas we would emphasize "believe." We believe Jesus of Nazareth has been exalted on high and was made by God both Lord and Christ. He is already seated on the throne and has poured forth the Holy Spirit. We believe in this reality and accept it as fact. The Spirit's outpouring is therefore the evidence of Jesus' exaltation; it is not the confirmation of our persistent prayer having been answered. The outpouring of the Holy Spirit is expressly linked to the exaltation of the Lord Jesus and not to our prayer or good deeds. Consequently, we should lift up the Lord, not ourselves: give glory to the Lord, not to ourselves: boast in the Lord, and not in ourselves.

3: Symptoms and Evidence of Receiving the Spirit's Outpouring*

Pentecost Does Not Literally Fulfill Joel's Prophecy

The story of Pentecost as recorded in the New Testament book of Acts does not fulfill the prophecy in the Old Testament book of Joel (2.28ff.). However, in a completely literal sense it does bear some—but only some—similarity to Joel. Unlike what is in Joel the events which occurred on the day of Pentecost contained no prophecy, no dream, and no vision. At Pentecost, there came a sound as of the rushing of a mighty wind and there were tongues that parted asunder like as in a fire (see Acts 2.1-3). Moreover, what was manifested in the disciples who were gathered at Pentecost was that they "began to speak with other tongues." But in the prophecy of Joel, there is no mentioning of such a sound nor of tongues. This is evidence that what happened on Pentecost is not a literal fulfillment of Joel's word, but is instead primarily that which runs along the same principle.

Some believers strongly affirm that to have the outpouring of the Holy Spirit, we must speak in tongues. But we know from the word of Peter that the experience of Pentecost is, as he said, that "this is that" which has been spoken through the prophet Joel (Acts 2.16). Peter said "this is that" and not "this fulfills that." These two expressions indicate mostly different principles. "Fulfill" conveys the idea of being literal; "is" conveys the idea of alikeness. Many consider this outpouring of the Holy Spirit at Pentecost as being the fulfillment of Joel's word, yet Joel made no mention of speaking in tongues. Many try to learn the technique of speaking in tongues, they even try

---

* Notes of message given at Chuenchow, Fukien Province, 19 November 1935.—Translator

to dream with dreams. But this is not what Peter had in mind. What Peter meant to say here is that the outpouring of the Holy Spirit which he witnessed is similar to that which Joel had prophesied. For this reason, we should not attempt to imitate the manifestation of the outpouring of the Holy Spirit that occurred on the day of Pentecost.

Manifestations Vary

The manifestations of the outpouring of the Holy Spirit are variable. Some may laugh, some may cry, some may sense power, and some may feel something upon them. We need to understand that these are what Peter referred to as "this is that" and not "this fulfills that." Some may sense being electrified, while others feel enwrapped by something. Some may leap, while others sit. All kinds of sensations are being experienced at the outpouring of the Holy Spirit. They constitute no problem in Peter's analysis of "this is that." Some people may seek the outpouring of the Holy Spirit and the result may be accompanied by tears and cries, but others may receive very different manifestations: for "this is that." Each has his own experience. We cannot say that because his experience is different from mine, therefore his is unreal. If a person receives a supernatural spirit and is able to say Jesus is Lord, then it is of God—irrespective of what its outward manifestation may be. Peter said "this is that," and so would we say "this is that." We must not imitate others, insisting upon our having the same manifestations.

Seek and Test

In the time of seeking for the outpouring of the Holy Spirit, you must test the spirit that falls upon you to see if this is of God (see 1 John 4.1). You should co-operate with God, never letting your mind become blank. Do not imitate others. Do not let your will be passive. Do not exert too much control nor let loose of all control. This is because evil spirits may counterfeit the Holy Spirit and give supernatural sensation and experience. The believer must test what he receives whether it is of the Holy Spirit or of the evil spirit. In order to distinguish the work of the Holy Spirit from the work of the evil spirit, we must first of all know their working principles. The Holy Spirit wants men to co-operate actively with Him, but the evil spirit looks for the passivity of man so as to manipulate him.

Consequently, in the process of seeking the outpouring of the Holy Spirit, we cannot afford to let our mind be blank and our will be passive. Passivity greatly delights the evil spirit. Trying to imitate others' experience also gives opportunity to the evil spirit to work. It is imperative that we practice that which we mentioned before: that we be actively working together with the Holy Spirit; and that we be watchful lest we be deceived. For it is possible for everyone to be deceived.

4: The Work of the Holy Spirit and the Benefits of Having His Outpouring*

The Work of the Holy Spirit

The Old and New Testaments show us that the work of the Holy Spirit is threefold: first, He gives people life; second, He dwells in people as life; and third, He falls upon people as power. These three include all the aspects of the work of the Holy Spirit. In Old Testament times there were only the first and the third of these aspects, but not the second. For at that time the Holy Spirit did not dwell in men. The difference between the Old and New Testaments lies in this second aspect, that is, in the indwelling of the Holy Spirit.

In the Old Testament period people might have received life; such as, for example, David, who had life. But there was also evidence of the outpouring of the Holy Spirit during that period, although it came upon only a chosen few such as the two artisans involved in the building of the tabernacle—Bezalel and Oholiab—who were "filled . . . with the Spirit of God, in wisdom," so as to be "skillful" in "all manner of workmanship" (Ex. 31.1-11). The Spirit of God was also upon Moses, and was evenly distributed upon the seventy elders (see Num. 11.16-25); the Spirit of God likewise fell upon the prophets, though many of the sons of the prophets—such as those of Elisha—did not have the Spirit falling upon them. There were altogether few in number who had the phenomenon with them. The book of the Judges, too, recorded some having the Spirit who were able to achieve things impossible to ordinary men. But like the prophets, the number was also quite small (see Judges 3.10, 6.34, 11.29, 13.25).

---

* Notes of message given at Chuenchow, Fukien Province, again on 19 November 1935.—Translator

During the opening period of the New Testament era, when the Lord was on earth, the Holy Spirit also fell upon certain people, such as Mary, Zacharias, John the Baptist, and the Lord himself. Nevertheless, at this time, but apart from the Lord Jesus, in whom the Holy Spirit had taken up His abode (see John 1.32-33), the Holy Spirit had not yet begun to dwell in men to be their life. Not until the time of Jesus' utterances about the Holy Spirit, as recorded in John 14.16-17, did the Holy Spirit begin to have a new work. Please notice the words "shall be" in verse 17, not "has been." For this will be a totally new aspect of His work. He is to "abide with you, and shall be in you." Unlike in the Old Testament period wherein the Holy Spirit did only the first and the third mentioned aspects of His work, here He begins a new work. He not only falls upon men to give them power, He also dwells in them.

Before His ascension, the Lord gave His disciples two great promises. The first He promised before His death, and the second He promised before His ascension. The first promise is that the Holy Spirit shall abide in the disciples (John 14.17). The second promise is that the Holy Spirit will come upon them (Acts 1.8). Thus, the Holy Spirit completes His threefold work. Because we are Gentiles, we may not realize the preciousness of this event. If we are Jews, though, we would know that the words "abide within" are quite marvelous, beyond our comprehension. Abraham, Isaac, Jacob, David, Solomon, Jeremiah, and so on—none of them had the Holy Spirit dwelling in them. The Old Testament merely stated that the Spirit of the Lord was upon them (see, for example, the case of David, in 1 Samuel 16.13). Only the New Testament speaks of the Holy Spirit as indwelling man. This is too wonderful a promise! "The word became flesh" is marvelous in our Lord's life. Now, later on, in us believers, the Spirit became flesh. How amazing this is!

When did the Holy Spirit begin to dwell in men? In John 14.17 we are told that the Lord said that the Holy Spirit "shall be in you." This word was spoken before His crucifixion. Then in John 20.22 we find that the Lord breathed on the disciples and said to them, "Receive ye the Holy Spirit." This happened after His resurrection. After the Lord was resurrected, the Holy Spirit came, and the disciples received the breathing of the Lord. The Holy Spirit is the breath of life of the Lord. Just as God breathed the breath of life into the nostrils of Adam after He had fashioned his body with the dust of the earth so that man became a living soul (see Gen. 2.7), so today the Lord breathes into us the Holy Spirit of life. Without the breathing of God into man, man was dead. So also, without such breathing of the Lord into the Church, the latter is likewise dead. This is the second aspect of the work of the Holy Spirit. Once we become familiar with the history of His work, we can interpret our present experience.

The promise of the Holy Spirit indwelling believers has its fulfillment on the day of the resurrection of the Lord. Forty days after His resurrection He further promised the disciples concerning the power of the Holy Spirit. On the day of Pentecost this promise of the Lord had its fulfillment. Comparing the two, which is better? In the Old Testament period the outpouring of the Holy Spirit was the special privilege of only some people—those such as the priests, prophets, judges, and so forth. Throughout the nation of Israel there might be only one person, either a king or some other special person, who possessed this blessing. The rest of the people had to go to him to hear his word. During Old Testament history such a person might appear but once in decades or in centuries. It was a very rare thing. But now in the New Testament time each and every one can have such an experience. This promise is so extraordinary that today all of us can possess it. This is indeed a special grace of the Lord. How joyful that we all may have the Holy Spirit coming upon us!

Before His ascension the Lord Jesus had commanded his disciples to wait in Jerusalem for the promised power from on

49

high (see Luke 24.49). By that time the disciples had already received the in dwelling life. They listened to the Lord and waited in prayer. Ten days later the day of Pentecost arrived and they were all filled with the Holy Spirit (see Acts 2.4). All who have read Acts 2 know that this speaks of the work of the Holy Spirit upon them. This is external. The Gospel according to Luke also speaks of the external work of the Holy Spirit upon men. It does not deal with His internal work. By comparing the Gospel according to John with the Gospel according to Luke and the book of Acts, we come to realize that the Holy Spirit works along two lines. One is that He works within men; the other is that He works on the outside of men.

Difference between Indwelling Spirit and Outpoured Spirit

The Holy Spirit indwelling man is for life, whereas the Holy Spirit upon man is for power. Unless we can distinguish these two aspects of work, we will not be able to understand the difference between the work of the Holy Spirit in the Old and in the New Testaments. The promise in the New Testament of the indwelling Holy Spirit is made by Christ before His death. This promised aspect of the Spirit's work is related to the death of the Lord and is fulfilled at the time of His resurrection. This work of the Holy Spirit within man is for the believer's life, for his daily living that he may bear those fruits of the Spirit such as holiness, righteousness, patience, joy, and so forth.

The promise of the Holy Spirit coming upon man is made by the Father in the Old Testament time and is reaffirmed by the Lord at His ascension. This aspect of the Holy Spirit is related to the ascension of the Lord and has its fulfillment at His ascension and exaltation. The Holy Spirit falls upon believers to clothe them with the Lord's power in being witnesses and in manifesting the gifts of the Spirit, thus having power to work for God and to accomplish His will.

4: The Work of the Holy Spirit
and the Benefits of Having His Outpouring

As we read the Old and New Testaments we must distinguish clearly between the Holy Spirit's work within men and upon men. Then shall we see that there is no contradiction in the many references to the work of the Holy Spirit. Otherwise, we will be puzzled by many seeming contradictions. According to God's word, each and every regenerated person must have the Holy Spirit indwelling him so that he also may receive the Spirit's outpouring. The one is "must"; the other is "may." Without any doubt, as soon as a person believes in the Lord, the Holy Spirit "must" dwell in him. On the other hand, he "may" also receive the outpouring of the Holy Spirit. By simply differentiating these two words you are able to see the wonder of it all.

Let me illustrate this. One day the Samaritans believed in the Lord and were baptized. The Bible does not say that they received both the indwelling and the outpouring of the Holy Spirit. Acts 8 records that these people had believed in the Lord and were baptized, but "as yet" the Holy Spirit "was fallen upon none of them" (v.16). So when the apostles in Jerusalem heard about it, they sent Peter and John to lay hands on the Samaritan believers so that they might receive the Holy Spirit. Now if a person is ignorant of the distinction between the indwelling and the outpouring of the Holy Spirit, he will find it difficult to explain this incident of the Samaritans who had believed and were baptized and yet had not received the Holy Spirit. Moreover, he will not know how to interpret certain passages in Romans 8, 1 John 4 and 1 Corinthians 6 in relation to this event. For all these passages indicate that as soon as one believes in the Lord that person has the Holy Spirit indwelling him. The fact of the matter is that the Samaritans did not lack the indwelling Spirit, they only lacked the outpoured Spirit.

The Holy Spirit Works Within and Without

The work of the Spirit within man is for life and living, enabling him to bear the fruit of the Holy Spirit. The work of the Spirit upon men is for witness and service, causing us to manifest spiritual gifts. Were a person to be filled with the Holy Spirit inwardly and have the Holy Spirit fall upon him outwardly, he would possess great power in serving the Lord. Yet if he is not filled within with the Holy Spirit and only receives outwardly the outpouring of the Spirit, he may be hurt instead of helped because he can easily become proud. For he who does not know the victorious life in his walk may receive the outpouring of the Holy Spirit, but a few months or years later, his spiritual condition will be exposed to everybody. Hence, we must experience both aspects of the Spirit's work.

The Holy Spirit Bears Witness Concerning Christ

The Holy Spirit does not bear witness to himself; He bears witness to Christ (see John 15.26). When a person sees the redemption of the cross he can be taught to ask the Holy Spirit to help him believe. This is to lead him to see Christ. As we talk about the work of the Holy Spirit in men, our attention is not on the Holy Spirit himself, because He bears witness concerning Christ. Even when we speak on the victorious life, we only mention how the Lord is resurrected to be our life; we do not focus on the Holy Spirit. For the latter's work is directly joined to Christ and His work. By seeing the work of Christ, people have the work of the Holy Spirit. By seeing the death of the Lord, they receive the regeneration of the Holy Spirit. By seeing the resurrection of the Lord, they have the Holy Spirit as their life. And when people see the ascended and enthroned Lord, they receive the outpouring of the Holy Spirit.

Not only the Spirit's outpouring witnesses to Christ, the Spirit's indwelling also testifies of Christ. On the one hand, the Holy Spirit in us gives us victory. On the other hand, the Holy

Spirit in us testifies that Christ is our all. The Holy Spirit in us enables us to bear the fruit of the Spirit (see Gal. 5.22-23), and such fruit is Christ in His entirety. For God has not given us the fruit of the Spirit in piecemeal fashion, such as a little love, a little joy, or a little patience, and so on. He gives us the total Christ. The fruit spoken of in Galatians 5.22 is presented to us as but one fruit, for in the original, the Greek word for fruit is cast in the singular number: having therefore the one fruit of the Holy Spirit, we have all the ingredients. It is not love without joy, or joy void of patience, etc. etc. God gives in wholesale fashion, not in retail. He gives us Christ. If we have love but not joy, this proves that it is our fruit and not the fruit of the Holy Spirit.

There are three chapters in the Bible which deal particularly with the Holy Spirit. These are found in 1 Corinthians 12-14: with chapters 12 and 14 speaking of the outpouring of the Holy Spirit—the Spirit without—and chapter 13 speaking of love, which bespeaks the Spirit within. We use "love" here to represent the fruit of the Spirit discussed in Galatians 5. This refers to the indwelling Spirit. The first ingredient of the fruit of the Spirit mentioned there is love, for without it nothing else counts—neither joy, nor peace, nor patience and so forth. Paul exhorts believers to seek after love, because with love they shall have all the above-mentioned qualities.

The Spirit Within More Important Than the Spirit Without

There is no comparison between the Spirit without and the Spirit within; that is to say, between the outpoured Holy Spirit and the indwelling Holy Spirit. For the outpouring of the Spirit cannot be deemed to be as essential as the indwelling Spirit. God had mercy on me in making me a minister, yet not for the outpouring of the Holy Spirit but for the victorious life; though in the ministry given me I also address the matter of the outpoured Spirit. The inward Spirit together with the outward Spirit is something tremendous. But to have the external outpouring minus the internal indwelling is dangerous. The best Christian walk is to have both the inward and the outward realities of the Spirit. Once having the inward ministry of the Spirit, one should seek the outward ministry of the Spirit. If there is not the inward Spirit, it is advisable to suspend temporarily the seeking of the outward Spirit.

In the Old Testament dispensation, after the priest had put the blood upon the tip of the right ear of him that was to be cleansed, upon the thumb of his right hand, and upon the great toe of his right foot, he followed by putting oil upon the same places (see Lev. 14.14-17). First he applied the blood, then he applied the oil. This means that the cross must first work upon your ear, hand and foot before the Holy Spirit can help you to walk and to work. The cross gets rid of your self, while the Holy Spirit comes to live for you. For the blood to be put on the ear, hand and foot means that the blood has blotted you out and thus removed you. But then the Holy Spirit comes to stand in as your ear, hand and foot. First, the victorious life, then the outpouring of the Holy Spirit. Accepting the application of the blood denotes co-death with Christ. And the work of the oil is to release the life of the Lord. Today, we expect the oil to fall upon our heads, yet having the outpouring of the oil before the working of the blood will only make us proud.

The saints in Corinth had the outward Spirit but not His inward fillings. They were carnal believers. Many have received the outpouring of the Holy Spirit, but within they are not full of life. In such people their lives have not changed. They live like the rest of the world. The outpouring of the Holy Spirit upon them is not linked to their inward life. A person most gifted without may not have a victorious life within. If a man's life is unclean, the Spirit's outside working will not cleanse him inside. But if a person has the proper life within plus the outpouring of the Spirit without, he can be a most useful man. In the entire records of the New Testament no local assembly seemed to have been worse than the church in Corinth. Nevertheless, Paul did not negate or attempt to blot out their outpouring of the Holy Spirit because of their inward immorality. He did not say that it was not good for the meeting there to have the outpouring of the Holy Spirit. He merely stated that due to confusion caused by outward gifts there needed to be some order. Though they were quite disorderly, Paul did not declare their condition to be attributable to the evil spirit. He advised them to do "all things decently and in order" (1 Cor. 14.40). This, too, must be our attitude. If some brothers and sisters among us show abnormal attitudes or manifestations, they need to be tested or helped to be orderly. We cannot judge them as outrightly wrong due to their so-called abnormalities.

Let me illustrate this. If someone should come to my room and see clothes scattered around in disarray, he cannot for this reason conclude that my clothes chest is not a chest and my clothes are not clothes. He can only say that these clothes are not tidily put away. Chaos can be restored to order. So that Paul only attempted to help set the Corinthian chaos and confusion in order. For example, he set right the order of speaking in tongues. If there was no interpreter, those who spoke in tongues were to keep quiet (see 1 Cor.14.28). Let the prophets speak one by one, he advised, at most letting two or three speak; and if there were more, let them keep silent and discern (see v.29).

First Corinthians 14 is therefore a setting in order; that is, how things should be arranged after the outpouring of the Holy Spirit has become a fact. Henceforth, we of today need to pay more attention to 1 Corinthians 14. On the one hand, we must learn to live victoriously; yet on the other hand, we must also seek the gifts of the Spirit. And thus we will maintain a balanced life.

Benefits of the Spirit's Outpouring

What benefits does the outpouring of the Holy Spirit bring to us? Since the Spirit's inward work is more essential, why do we need this outward work of outpouring? We ought to realize that if those who know the Person of the Holy Spirit indwelling within and who live a holy life were to receive the outpouring of the Holy Spirit as well, this would enable them to share their inner holiness with others. We know many people who are rich inwardly, but they are unable to supply to others what is within them. Men may admire them and respect them, but they cannot receive help from them because the latter lack the outpouring of the Holy Spirit. Let us therefore consider what practical profits can result from the Spirit's outpouring.

1. Grants the power to communicate. The outpouring of the Holy Spirit gives you the power to communicate, that is to say, to channel forth what is in you to others. People who have learned much before God and yet lack the power to share with others are enabled to distribute the riches inside themselves once they do receive the outpouring of the Spirit. Yet those who only have the indwelling Holy Spirit can be likened to a power house whose impact upon its surroundings is minimal: there may be much light in the power house; nevertheless, the entire city lies in darkness. In order to channel light to the city there must be power lines to connect the power house with the city. If, of course, there is nothing in the power house, the connection of power lines is absolutely useless. But even if there is something in the power house, it is still useless without the power lines. In this illustration, of course, the outpouring of the Holy Spirit can be likened to the power lines. Is it not absurd that many Christians have numerous power lines and yet they use candle lights in the night because they have nothing in them? They may think of communicating something to others, but they have nothing inside them to communicate. They are useless. Consequently, we need to be filled both within and without. By knowing the victorious life we have something inside, and by seeking the outpouring of the Holy Spirit we have the power to give of that inward life.

2. *Instills courage.* Some people have riches within, but they are very timid. They have to deliberate and resolve many times over before they can give testimonies. Others may have really believed in the Lord Jesus, yet they are afraid to distribute gospel tracts. For those who have not yet received the outpouring of the Holy Spirit or who are afraid of such an experience, may I challenge you by asking if you are as bold as those brethren who have had the outpouring of the Holy Spirit? You may have something inside you, but you are timid. Others may not have your riches, yet they are not afraid—a trait of boldness which you do not have. I do not encourage those who are already into the outpouring of the Holy Spirit to go on a rampage; nevertheless, I do exhort those who for the first time have this experience to proceed immediately to bear witness to it because they who were formerly timid have now been given courage.

Brethren who have received the outpouring of the Holy Spirit can be grouped into two categories: one category of people are thin-skinned and still timid; the other category of people are thick-skinned and unafraid. Before I received the outpouring of the Holy Spirit I would sometimes follow a gospel friend for one or two miles but dared not witness to him. I had the courage to pray and to read the Bible on the train, but I had to exert some effort to distribute gospel tracts. Once I had received the outpouring of the Holy Spirit, however, I did not care anymore about the way I dressed (see below, at point 3) and I had great boldness. I could now be classified as not only being thick-skinned but as having no skin as well!

3. *Removes self-consciousness.* Self-consciousness is bad for Christians. A self-conscious person is aware of his clothing,

whether good or bad; he is sensitive to people's reaction. When invited to eat out, he finds no liberty to preach the gospel to his host. When he meets a newcomer, he cannot talk to him unless he has first carefully prepared himself. These conditions exist because he always is conscious of himself. He can pray by himself in the room, but he cannot pray as freely in public as he can in his room. Before the public he has to change his tone, words and attitude for fear of displeasing men. These symptoms indicate deep self-consciousness. Such a person's spirit is encircled by the soul, and thus he is not free.

Once there was a meeting in a brother's sitting room. The Holy Spirit was poured forth at the meeting; everybody was set free. Such freedom is not license, but liberty of the spirit. Sometimes in a gathering, people are so cautious that no one dares to speak. God used Evan Roberts to save many souls. Many testified that he was the one person in the world who had no self-consciousness. He could laugh when he felt to laugh. He could look at people when he wanted to do so. Only a person devoid of self-consciousness can work for God. To be delivered from self-consciousness we need the outpouring of the Holy Spirit, for by it we are set free.

4. Changes the atmosphere. A man filled with the Holy Spirit can change the atmosphere. A room may be quiet, but when someone enters in, immediately it becomes noisy. Or the room is noisy, but at his entrance it suddenly becomes quiet. What was quiet becomes noisy, and what was noisy becomes quiet. A person such as this can affect the room atmosphere. Our failure to have an impact lies in our inability to bring in a spiritual atmosphere. We simply follow what others are doing. We cannot influence them, but are influenced by them. But a person who has the outpouring of the Holy Spirit is able to turn the atmosphere in accordance with his atmosphere. May we all receive the outpouring of the Holy Spirit so that we may be atmosphere-changers!

5. Can have the power to work. In our receiving the outpouring of the Holy Spirit we can ask for spiritual gifts and the power to work. We have no power without the outpouring of the Holy Spirit, but with it we come into possession of the power to work for God. This makes a great difference. If we are to have power to serve, we must have the outpouring of the Holy Spirit.

Some Questions and Answers

Question: Can the indwelling Spirit be visible to others as is the outpoured Spirit?

Answer: When you believe in the Lord, you receive the indwelling Spirit. This you know, though it is unknown to other people. The Holy Spirit indwelling us is the work of God. He cannot be seen by men. But when the Holy Spirit falls upon man, people can readily see the manifestations thereof.

Question: Does Acts 8 mention the Holy Spirit indwelling men?

Answer: No, it only makes reference to the Holy Spirit coming upon men.

Question: Acts 19 records the twelve saints in Ephesus who had received the baptism of John yet had never even heard of the coming of the Holy Spirit. When Paul arrived there, he questioned them whether they had received the Spirit when they believed. They answered, "Nay, we did not so much as hear whether the Holy Spirit was given" (v.2). Would they perish in their present condition?

Answer: Theological students might answer "they would perish," for they had not yet heard about, or received, the Holy Spirit. Therefore, at that moment they must be considered

59

among the lost. But I say, they were saved, they would not have perished. You might ask, then, how they could be saved without their having the Holy Spirit. Well, we know they already had faith. Paul merely pointed out to them that the baptism of John they had earlier received was inadequate because it was only "the baptism of repentance, [John] saying unto the people that they should believe on him that should come after him, that is, on Jesus" (v.4). That was why they had not received the Holy Spirit and not because they had not believed on Jesus. Indeed, Paul did not even raise the issue of faith in the Lord Jesus with them. No, what these Ephesians lacked was the Spirit's outpouring, not the Spirit's indwelling of Romans 8. Furthermore, the record of Acts reckons these twelve as disciples (see 19.1b). During those days believers were disciples, and disciples were believers (cf. Acts 11.26c). Such were saved people. Hence, what these twelve at Ephesus lacked was the coming of the Holy Spirit upon them; they did not lack the Holy Spirit indwelling them.

Let me illustrate it this way. Several decades ago you and I believed in the Lord and thus received the Holy Spirit to dwell in us. Later on, we came to know and experience tongues and prophecies—the outpouring of the Holy Spirit. The indwelling of the Holy Spirit does not need the speaking in tongues, prophecies or the other gifts as evidence. It cannot be said that because you and I do not have these evidences of the outpouring of the Holy Spirit that we do not have the Holy Spirit. On the contrary, the Holy Spirit has been dwelling in us ever since the time we had believed and received the Lord Jesus.

Question: How important is it to distinguish between the inward and outward works of the Holy Spirit?

Answer: On the one hand, people with the inward Spirit who yet lack the outward Spirit cannot be easily recognized; on the other hand, people with the outward Spirit who lack

60

something of the inward working of the Spirit can quickly be deceived. The latter category of people can fall into boasting about how they are able to win many souls—they even boasting over the number of souls they have saved—and claiming that they have no need of receiving advice from anyone. Such proud words come out of the mouth of one who has received the outpouring of the Holy Spirit but who is very much lacking in a further work of the indwelling Holy Spirit. For this reason, we must pay more attention to the inward work of the Holy Spirit than to His outward work.

Appendix:
Difference between Regeneration and Filling

1. Regeneration relates to initial salvation, while filling relates to victory thereafter.

2. Regeneration is associated with life, whereas filling is associated with living.

3. Regeneration is connected with justification, while filling is connected with sanctification.

4. Regeneration gives to the believer in Christ a new life other than the old life in Adam, whereas filling gives increase of that new life through the repeated infillings of the Holy Spirit in the believer.

5. Regeneration in a believer is the work of the Holy Spirit that is based on Jesus' substitutionary death on the cross, while filling is the filling of the Holy Spirit in the human spirit for implementing or working out in the believer all the meanings of the cross.

6. Regeneration speaks of the commencement of life, whereas filling speaks of the maturation of life.

5: Further Talk on the Spirit's Outpouring*

1. Concerning those who have received the outpouring of the Holy Spirit.

After receiving the Spirit's outpouring you daily need to control your spirit. God is not a God of confusion, but of peace. So, you must learn to obey God and not overly let loose of your spirit. In this matter, you are responsible not to lose control of your spirit. The outpouring of the Holy Spirit is not for amusement. Do not ask for the outpouring if the need for it is not present. Once a brother in Chefoo received the outpouring of the Holy Spirit. Then, while at mealtime he again experienced an outpouring. Since there was no need, he later on refused it. On another occasion—this time while he was on a train—he experienced a further outpouring which he declined, for there was no need at that moment. He was most powerful in winning difficult souls. He was right in following the principle that the outpouring of the Holy Spirit is to be sought after only in time of need and not to be treated as an object of amusement or for spiritual enjoyment.

When a person receives the Spirit's outpouring for the first time, I believe it most likely is genuine. I cannot be so certain of his later experiences. Jesus declared to His disciples: "If ye then, being evil, know how to give good gifts unto your children, how much more shall your heavenly Father give the Holy Spirit to them that ask him?" (Luke 11.13) If we stand on this scripture verse and ask, what we will be given by God is the Holy Spirit. Many ask God for the outpouring of the Spirit with improper motives—such as, a desire to satisfy their curiosity, to show their superiority or spirituality, and so forth.

---

* Notes of message given at Chuenchow, Fukien Province, 26 November 1935.—Translator

And thus, the evil spirit is given ground to counterfeit. We therefore need to be very cautious in this matter. Never ask for the outpouring of the Holy Spirit out of curiosity or to be amused. Ask only when there is a definite need.

On the other hand, concerning the testing of the spirits, we must at all times test the spirit whenever there is any kind of outpouring. We have to test each time because we are no match for the evil one in the spiritual realm.

2. Must not rely on the Spirit's outpouring more than on prayer and faith.

In our working for God we must not rely on the outpouring of the Holy Spirit more than on prayer and faith. In God's work, prayer and faith are absolute necessities. The Spirit's outpouring gives us power; nonetheless, we should not desire after it as a shortcut. Prayer and faith cannot be substituted for by the outpouring of the Holy Spirit. In a meeting for the seeking of the outpouring, many may outrageously let loose of themselves. They think the more they let go, the more spiritual they become. This will result in many problems. We ought to realize that for the Holy Spirit to be released His working must begin from our inner spirit, pass through our soul, and reach to our body.

It is therefore most dangerous for a person to receive the outpouring of the Holy Spirit without first having the dealings of the cross within. In experiencing the Spirit's outpouring, what one receives is first the power of the Holy Spirit, and then it is released together with the strength of the soul and the energy of the body. And hence there is the danger that if a believer has not been dealt with by the cross, the release of the Holy Spirit's power will result in an impure amalgam as it passes through that person's undealt-with soul and body. Indeed, this process can be likened to how clean underground water passing through the various strata in the earth eventually flows forth as unclean water.

How do we distinguish whether or not it is the power of the outpoured Spirit that is being manifested? We can test it by means of the cross. The life of the body and soul needs to be dealt with by the cross; and then, at the outpouring of the Holy Spirit, what is released is only the power of the Spirit. But if the life of the body and soul has not been dealt with by the cross, then the energies of soul and body will be released at the outpouring of the Holy Spirit. Here, therefore, we can discover an acid test: when a person is free and loses control, what will he do? The one whose bodily energy has not been properly dealt with by the cross will discharge its power at the outpouring of the Holy Spirit. The same is true of the soul. If the person's soul has not been dealt with, his soul power will be released.

May I speak seriously to my fellow-workers that they must especially guard against the release of their soul power. The weaker the physical strength, the easier will be the release of the latent power of the soul.* For those who have been dealt with by the cross, however, they can detect in a meeting for the outpouring of the Holy Spirit exactly what soul power is being released and from where. Someone may mislead a thousand unknowledgeable people, but he cannot deceive the one who has been dealt with by the cross.

The Bible mentions two kinds of power: one is the power of resurrection (see Phil. 3.21), which is inside of us. The other is the power of the Holy Spirit which is outside of us, and is the power manifested at the Spirit's outpouring. If there is the power of the Holy Spirit without but not the power of resurrection within, the power of the soul and body will also be

---

* For a much more thorough discussion of this subject, the reader can consult Watchman Nee, The Latent Power of the Soul (New York: Christian Fellowship Publishers, 1972). Originally published in Chinese in issues of Revival magazine, 1932, but now translated into English.—Translator

released at the release of the power of the Holy Spirit. Those with experience can discern these two streams. This is not what we seek. We want only one stream, that of the absolutely pure Spirit.

We must also know what the resurrection life is. Resurrection life is the power of living again. "Living again" signifies that power which has already passed through death. All the natural goodness in us—such as the power, affection and influence of the soul—must go through death. In a meeting, those who have been dealt with by the cross can supply others with a pure spiritual supply. The life they give is pure. There is not a mixture in it of soul or flesh.

In China there was a servant of God. He was a dear brother. He was very powerful and was used to win many souls. One day I saw him pour oil on the heads of thirty or forty people. He struck their faces, even kicked them. Yet they were all healed. No one should ever say that this was the result of the evil spirit. For no doubt about it, this brother had the power of the outpoured Spirit upon him; but he did not have the power of resurrection life within him. And hence there were these uncrucified behaviors present during this healing service. The outpouring of the Holy Spirit gives a blessed power, and the working of the cross purifies this power as it passes through the human vessel. For the cross stands against the old creation: with the cross the old creation is set aside. So that when those who have been dealt with by the cross do the work of God, they have the power of resurrection within and the power of the Holy Spirit without. As a consequence, though today we are talking mainly about the Spirit's outpouring, we must not lay aside the truth of the cross heretofore mentioned. For this truth of the cross is most essential because it alone can enable the believer to walk in a clean path.

In helping brothers and sisters, we must be sure that we first help them to experience the victorious life and then lead them to seek the outpouring of the Holy Spirit. This advice should never be reversed, for having the power of the outpoured Spirit without also having the resurrection power within is dangerous. Before a person receives the Spirit's outpouring, we should tell him to exert a certain degree of control lest he become totally disengaged. We must teach the brethren how to cooperate with the Holy Spirit. Until people can cooperate with Him we must teach them the basic truth.

3. The difference between the outpouring and the infilling of the Holy Spirit.

Let us look again at the difference between the outpouring and the infilling of the Holy Spirit. The outpouring is for all the saints, whereas the infilling is for a special group of people: those who have emptied themselves. While studying the Bible, we should notice the contrasting connection there is between words. For example: resurrection is linked with death, filling with emptying. By bringing related words together we come to the accurate knowledge of a given word. People who are filled with the Holy Spirit are those who have emptied themselves, for filling is linked to emptying. Before Pentecost, one hundred and twenty disciples were assembled at one place. They all received the outpouring as well as the infilling of the Holy Spirit because they had been dealt with by the risen Lord (see Acts 2.2, 3-4). For this reason, they could gather for ten days and pray with one accord. The three thousand on the day of Pentecost also received the outpouring of the Holy Spirit, but the Scriptures did not say that they had experienced the Spirit's filling. The one hundred and twenty had both the outpouring and the infilling, whereas the three thousand had only the outpouring. Later on, another five thousand received the outpouring of the Holy Spirit, but they too had not received the filling of the Holy Spirit.

How do we know that the three thousand and the five thousand received only the outpouring and not the infilling of the Holy Spirit? Because in the church at that time, if all the people had been filled with the Holy Spirit, the problem of daily ministration could not have arisen. But "there arose a murmuring of the Grecian Jews against the Hebrews, because their widows were neglected in the daily ministration" (Acts 6.1). This incident proves that these disciples were not filled with the Holy Spirit. Due to this problem, the apostles appointed seven to serve tables. These seven, we are told, were all persons full of the Holy Spirit (see v.3). Had the entire congregation been filled with the Holy Spirit, the infilling would have been so pervasive among these new believers that there would have been no need to choose. But because of the fact that not all among these many thousand believers were filled with the Holy Spirit, there needed to be the choosing of the seven. This proves that though many at that time had experienced the outpouring of the Holy Spirit, they had not had the infilling of the Holy Spirit.

As regards the Spirit's outpouring, the ascended Lord pours forth the Holy Spirit upon us because of our faith. Yet it has little relationship to life. But with respect to the filling of the Holy Spirit, it is the risen Lord who infills us because of our obedience. It requires a holy life in us.

If you want to be filled with the Holy Spirit you must empty yourself: you must be hungry and unsatisfied. Only in this way can you be inwardly filled and satisfied. There must always be an emptying, always a hungering. Then you can always be filled with the Holy Spirit. Never accept what you have already received as being sufficient. To the contrary, let the cross work daily in your life so as to be daily filled. The moment you fail to live victoriously, at that moment you forfeit the infilling of the Holy Spirit. Today you are filled with the Holy Spirit because you experience the dealing and emptying of the cross and live a victorious life.

Once I was having a meal in a brother's house. I finally decided I had eaten enough. But that brother continued to add food to my plate, and not just once or twice but twenty-odd times. I thought to myself, When will he stop adding? Now this is just the way it is for us in the state of grace. For the supply of God is always something to be experienced more and more. In God's grace, it is a matter of grace upon grace, an abundance of His grace. The more we experience victory, the more we are filled with the Holy Spirit. We are to be filled numberless times. But we must never reach the point of being content with what we have received, for the Holy Spirit can fill us more and more. The measure of the first filling is different from that of the second, the second from the third, the third from the fourth, and so on. The deeper you are dug into by the cross, the fuller you shall be filled with the Holy Spirit. The deeper the cut by the cross, the greater the filling of the Holy Spirit. Sometimes your heart may ache, sometimes your trials may be too much to bear, sometimes you feel it is impossible to run the course. These are the crosses which keep burrowing down through you in order to enlarge your capacity to make you fuller and richer.

Under such circumstances, do not be afraid of shedding tears or of having the heart wounded. If you can bear the digging up and the burrowing down, you will be used of the Lord. But if you fret and have controversy with God, you at once lose your victorious life and any outpouring of the Holy Spirit will be of no help. Therefore, be before the Lord and let His cross pierce deeply and cut you. Each cutting of the cross severs something from you that you love and long for. These cuttings are the work of the cross for the increase of your measure of grace. The greater your capacity, the more the grace.

Someone may consider himself as having already been cut and wounded by the cross and filled with the Holy Spirit. Actually, however, he is as a mere shell that is filled with water; such cannot yet be termed true affliction nor a real filling. When we are confronted with things that are opposite to our wish, they can enlarge us the most if handled properly. Each time we submit ourselves under the will of God in such matters and allow the cross to cut us, we give opportunity to the Holy Spirit to fill us once more.

4. What is required of us in giving testimony.

We need to be a sanctified people before sinners as well as before professing Christians. Unless we experience the cross and are filled with the Holy Spirit, our testimony before men will be weak and incomplete. We should let people know the centrality of God as well as the full counsel of God. We should let them see that we have offered ourselves up to God to fulfill His will. We seek for God's ultimate purpose and not just to testify to minor truths.

Do not freely auction up your life of victory. Having been poured upon by the Holy Spirit, you should testify more as to how the Lord delivers you from sin and lives for you. This will create a hunger in people's heart. If your service is to be effective, you must stir up the desire of the people. As you are led of God, you should clearly tell them how the Lord becomes your victorious life and you should help them to empty themselves for the filling of the Holy Spirit.

There is yet another matter you should pay special attention to; which is, that you should not treat the outpouring of the Holy Spirit as something of a curiosity that is to be propagated everywhere you go. Only when you are led by the Lord should you testify to it. If a person has a need for the outpouring of the Holy Spirit, take him to your Lord, gather a few, and then pray together till he receives the Spirit's outpouring.

6: Still More on the Spirit's Work and His Outpouring*

A. The Work of the Holy Spirit

We find that in the Old Testament times the Holy Spirit provided people with new life; yet we find the same work being done by the Holy Spirit in the New Testament period: the granting of new life. So that with respect to this matter of new life, both the Old and New Testaments agree, all occurrences of life-giving work included therein having been that of the Holy Spirit. Let us never think that the granting of new life is a specialty to be found only in the New Testament. The Lord told Nicodemus (who at that moment was still under the Old Testament dispensation) that he being the teacher of Israel ought to have understood the new birth of which He was then speaking (see John 3.10). This is therefore strong evidence that those in the Old Testament era must have been conversant about this matter of life, too.

What, then, is the basic difference between the work of the Holy Spirit in the Old Testament period and in the New? What can we say is the special work of the Holy Spirit found in the New Testament which sets it apart from the Old Testament? One thing which is certain about this matter in the Old Testament is, that we never find being mentioned that the Holy Spirit dwelt in men. Yes, there is no doubt that during those earlier times He worked in human hearts, but He never took up His abode there. We cannot find a single verse in the Old Testament which states that the Holy Spirit dwelt in man. We do indeed read about the Holy Spirit falling upon men, but not about His dwelling in them. In relation to the Spirit, the Old

---

* Notes of message given at Shanghai, sometime during 1938-1942, a more exact date unobtainable.—Translator

Testament scriptures always use the word *epi*—which is "upon"—and never use the word *en*—which is "in." In the New Testament, we still see mentioned the Holy Spirit falling upon men. He indeed continues to do this kind of work, but He does far more in this new era. As the moment for the Lord's betrayal approached, Jesus said: "he [the Holy Spirit] abideth with you, and shall be in you" (John 14.17c). This is a totally new work. Henceforth, the New Testament scriptures will speak of man as the temple of the Holy Spirit, which means that the Holy Spirit dwells in men.

Therefore, we see in the New Testament era the twofold work of the Holy Spirit: (1) He comes upon men; (2) He dwells in men. His coming upon men is still for power, for doing miracles, and for witnessing. His dwelling in men is for sanctification. In dwelling in us, the Holy Spirit supplies Christ to us to be our life and to enable us to bear the fruit of holiness.

By carefully distinguishing the above-mentioned twofold work of the Holy Spirit, we come to realize that certain concepts about the Holy Spirit are erroneous. Many consider all their problems solved if they experience their own "Pentecost." But now that they have had their Pentecost, is their problem of sanctification being resolved? Does it help them to overcome their temper? No, it has not settled this matter of overcoming sin. For Pentecost can only bestow gifts, not fruits.

When Paul looked at the condition of the church in Corinth, he did not say, "The situation here is so bad that we must stop everything." Many teachers would cast the Corinthian church out because of all the carnal things present there. Not so with Paul; he brought in something to balance the Corinthian believers: "Know ye not that ye are a temple of God, and that the Spirit of God dwelleth in you?" (1 Cor. 3.16) In essence he told them they needed to learn what was meant by the Holy Spirit dwelling in men.

These teachers would also teach us, saying: "Gifts are kindergarten stuff. We are now grown-ups. We do not need to play with things such as tongues. Our faith has made much progress. We are more advanced than the apostles. So we will throw all these things away." On the other hand, too many of those who advocate the gifts of the Holy Spirit think that aside from gifts there is nothing more, they ignoring the importance of the development of the inward life. They despise people who have not had the same experience as they; namely, that of the outpoured Spirit. They boastfully declare, "On such and such a day, I received the baptism of the Holy Spirit." Both of these concepts are wrong: the word of God indeed saying, "forbid not to speak with tongues" (1 Cor.14.39b); and it also saying, "moreover a most excellent way show I unto you" (1 Cor. 12.31b)—which is the way of love that is introduced in the verse immediately thereafter (13.1) and fully discussed in what follows in this now famous "love chapter" of the Bible.

In the New Testament we see the two sides of the Holy Spirit. From about the time of the Lord's last supper with His disciples to the day of Pentecost the Bible mentions the Holy Spirit four times: (1) at around the time of the Last Supper Jesus spoke of the Holy Spirit as the Comforter: "I will pray the Father, and he shall give you another Comforter, . . . for he . . . shall be in you" (John 14.16-17); (2) after the Last Supper the first mention of the Holy Spirit occurred on the evening of the Lord's resurrection. Jesus breathed on the disciples and said to them, "Receive ye the Holy Spirit" (John 20.22b); (3) before His ascension the Lord said, "Behold, I send forth the promise of my Father upon you: but tarry ye in the city, until ye be clothed with power from on high" (Luke 24.49); and (4) the Holy Spirit came on the day of Pentecost (Acts 2.1-4).

The belief is commonly accepted that the promise of the Comforter was fulfilled on the day of Pentecost, but this interpretation is not according to the word of God. John wrote John 14, but he also wrote John 20. In Chapter 14 the Lord is recorded as promising that "the Father ... shall give you another Comforter" (v.16). Then in Chapter 20, that promise is shown to have been fulfilled. Before the death of the Lord there is no mention in the Scriptures of the promise of the Holy Spirit coming upon men. No, before His death the Lord had only promised that the Holy Spirit would dwell in men. Then, on the day of His resurrection, He breathed on His disciples and said, "Receive ye the Holy Spirit" (20.22). What is breath? Breath is life. If we cease to breathe, we cease to live. Christ breathed on His disciples and said, "Receive ye the Holy Spirit."

Now did the Lord also say to His disciples at this time, "You must wait for fifty days"? No, He breathed on them; and there and then they received the Holy Spirit. So John 14 was fulfilled in John 20. The promise made at about the time of the Last Supper was fulfilled on the day of the Lord's resurrection. Only after forty days further had passed did the Lord say to His disciples, "Tarry ye in the city, until ye be clothed with power from on high" (Luke 24.49). Hence Pentecost was the fulfillment of Luke 24, the final chapter of that Gospel. Both the Gospel of Luke and the book of Acts are written by Luke; and therefore, the material in Acts 1 can be reckoned as Chapter 25 of Luke, for it is a continuation of Luke's Gospel. Acts is but Luke's continued narration of events. This would only be natural.

From all the above we can see that the indwelling Holy Spirit is given by the breathing of the Lord. It is based on His resurrection and is for life. That Spirit that comes upon me comes through the glorification of the Lord, and it is for service.

B. The Outpouring of the Holy Spirit

In our consideration together today we would like to inquire into four different passages of Scripture that have to do with the outpouring of the Holy Spirit. From each one and from all of them together we can perhaps draw a few conclusions and derive some spiritual principles which can help us to better understand, appreciate and experience this aspect of our Christian walk.

Acts 2.32-41. In reading this section of Acts 2 we must pay special attention to verse 33: "he hath poured forth this, which ye see and hear." On the day of Pentecost the Lord Jesus had poured forth the Holy Spirit. What is this pouring forth based upon? A careful reading of this entire passage will reveal that it is based on the exaltation of Jesus! It is not because of our clean heart or our earnest seeking and fervent prayer, but because of Christ having been highly exalted: "Let all the house of Israel therefore know assuredly, that God hath made Jesus both Lord and Christ" (v.36). The outpouring of the Spirit did not occur to prove man's goodness and sincerity but to prove to all the house of Israel that Jesus is Lord and Christ. How does God prove this? The "therefore" in verse 36 connects with verse 33. What did they see and hear? It was the Holy Spirit being poured forth. The outpouring of the Spirit of God is the evidence of the Lordship of Jesus (cf. John 7.39).

The Spirit has already been poured forth. This is the gospel. One day, after I had explained this truth to a person in Christ, he knelt down and prayed, "Lord Jesus, You have received from the Father two things: glory is for You yourself, and the Spirit is for me. You have already been glorified, but I have not yet had the Spirit." Then he quickly corrected himself and said, "It is not possible for anyone to say that You have not been glorified. Likewise, it is also impossible to say that I have not had the Spirit." Immediately the Holy Spirit came upon him.

Forgiveness of sins is based on the finished work of Christ on the cross. The outpouring of the Spirit of Christ is based on His being on the throne. This is to say that the outpouring of His Spirit is based on His glorification (compare again John 7.39). The condition for the outpouring of the Spirit, therefore, is His glorification, and not my being and doing. I have not done anything to have my sins forgiven, so I need not do anything to receive the Spirit. Let us read verse 38 of Acts 2, which says: "Repent ye, and be baptized every one of you in the name of Jesus Christ unto the remission of your sins; and ye shall receive the gift of the Holy Spirit." The condition for receiving that spiritual gift is the same condition for receiving the forgiveness of sins. By fulfilling the condition for the forgiveness of God, we also fulfill the condition for receiving the Spirit. If I go to the store, pay ten dollars for two books and take away only one book, need I—in going back for the other book—again pay ten dollars?

Acts 8.14-17. This passage relates how the Spirit fell upon the Samaritan believers. People may be saved individually, such as in the case of the robber on the cross. But the outpouring of the Holy Spirit in the present case is not for the individual member; instead it is for the whole body of Christ. For the outpouring is given to unite all the scattered members into one Body. It is like cement that unites the separated stones into a single construction, "for in one Spirit were we all baptized into one body" (1 Cor.12.13a). In the case of the Samaritans, Philip had not gone out to Samaria as one sent out by the Church. If the Holy Spirit had fallen upon the Samaritans at the time of Philip's preaching to them, the oneness of the body of Christ would have been lost. The apostles from Jerusalem therefore came and laid hands on them, a procedure thus demonstrating their unity with them. This expressed the oneness of the body of Christ, and so the Holy Spirit immediately fell upon the Samaritans. Thus right from the commencement of Church history, God revealed the principle of order. The Samaritans were saved all right, but they had not yet experienced the fellowship of the Body. This principle must be established before the Holy Spirit could be poured forth.

Acts 10.44-48. "While Peter yet spake these words, the Holy Spirit fell on all them that heard the word." If, as He had done to the Samaritans, God had had Peter lay hands on these Gentiles gathered in the house of Cornelius as their way of receiving the Spirit instead of letting the Spirit fall directly upon them, would Peter have been willing to do so? The laying on of hands implies union, recognition. Would he as a staunch Jewish believer have recognized these Gentile hearers of the gospel? Even if he had laid hands on them and the Spirit had come down, how would the Christian brethren in Jerusalem have reacted? They would have said to Peter, "This is all your fault. If you had not laid hands on the Gentiles, this thing would not have happened!" They would most likely have held on to their Jewish viewpoint. As it turned out, Peter did not lay hands on those who gathered in Caesarea at the house of Cornelius the Roman centurion. He had not even mentioned the Spirit in his message. Yet while he was still speaking, the Spirit fell upon all of them. Consequently, Peter could boldly say, "Can any man forbid the water, that these [Gentiles] should not be baptized, who have received the Holy Spirit as well as we [Jews]?" Because the Holy Spirit had indeed come down, what could Peter say?

Acts 19.1-6. The coming down of the Holy Spirit on this subsequent occasion is to reinforce further what had happened earlier at Caesarea. For on both occasions the outpouring fell upon the Gentiles. These here at Ephesus were true believers because (1) in verse 1 they are referred to as "disciples," a term synonymous with Christians (see 11.26); and (2) if they were not already truly saved, then Paul could have been accused of preaching baptismal regeneration. Paul baptized them in the name of the Lord Jesus. By this they bore witness to the fact that they were united with the Head. And the laying on of hands immediately followed thereafter to testify to the fact that they were united with the whole body of Christ.

The above four passages of Scripture prove that the outpouring of the Holy Spirit upon believers is what the whole Body enjoys together. They also point to the power of ministry that was so much evident in these early servants of God. Why is it that there are so few today with real power? It is because most are lacking in the incorporating work of the cross in their lives. Having the "inside" Spirit as well as the "outside" Spirit results in power that was so evident in the ministry of these earlier ministers of the gospel. Paul talked much about the power of the resurrection of Christ. Without experiencing the inward resurrection life, there can be no real power. Resurrection is that life which enters into death and comes forth again, with all natural power having been eliminated. We possess natural strength, intelligence, personality and other facets of our undealt-with soul power. These must be cast aside before there can be the power of resurrection. All which does not come through regeneration must be let go. "That which is born of the flesh is flesh" (John 3.6). How we depend so much on our natural strength to do sacred works! With our own earthly eloquence, we miss out on having divinely spiritual utterance. How we need a turning. We need to have revelation, to see the hatefulness and vanity of all these natural powers. God has no use for our natural power and wisdom, and many other soulish things.

7. The Holy Spirit and the Law*

We believers ought to live by the Holy Spirit, not by the law. Many do not know what the law is, hence they are equally ignorant of what the Holy Spirit is. They know neither what it means to live by the law nor what it means to live by the Spirit. Moreover, the reason for our failure in God's work is due to our working by the law and not by the Holy Spirit. Working according to the law gives no power nor spiritual result, for law deals with judgment.

What the Law Is

The Old Testament law is not limited to just the Ten Commandments but also to the hundreds of rules and statutes that were subsequently given. All of them together constitute the Old Testament law. The children of Israel in the Old Testament period had the law. But so does the Church of the New Testament have law (see later below).

What is really the principle of the law? The law is God's will inscribed on stone or written on paper, from one to thousands of articles. If people keep these thousands of precepts, they will be able to distinguish good from evil, right from wrong. They will know where they should go and not go, what they ought to do and not do. This is the law, and it is the law of death. When people conduct themselves according to such dead law, they put God behind their backs. Such a situation can be likened to a student who is able to keep the rules of his school without ever having to see the school principal for a whole month. This is what the law is. All matters pointing to right and wrong, good and evil are made known through the written-out law. All are kept intelligently—that is, by the

---

* Notes of message given at Chuenchow, Fukien Province, 20 November 1935.—Translator

mind—and not by means of the guidance of the God who dwells deep within. Such is the keeping of the law.

Like the student mentioned above and his school principal, many have the knowledge of good and evil, right and wrong without ever having to have any communion with God. Such knowledge is useless, and such people are under the law. By this principle, you can understand how many things are done under the law. Men love the law because it causes them to know right and wrong quite easily. Most people are afraid of living by the Spirit; they prefer to live according to certain rules. Although keeping the law is something rigid and dead, it is nonetheless also easy, for you are able to know how many articles you have kept and which article you have lacked observing. The law leads people away from God, for with it men can leave God outside without having to draw near to Him. But we who know Christ as life should never live again under the law: we must live by the newness of the Holy Spirit (see Rom. 7.6).

Living under the Law

Let us now discuss what walking according to the law is. It was not until a few years ago—that is, in 1928—that I began to see what keeping the law means. I had been a preacher for some years, yet I did not know what it was. So far as theological knowledge was concerned, I could expound it. But I did not know it in practical experience. During that year, which was after the Lord had healed me of a very serious sickness, I was recuperating at a beach and I met Simon Meek. We lived there together. His health was also poor and he asked for my help. I asked him wherein I could help, and he answered that he could be helped if I could tell him whether divine healing was scriptural. I told him that God was most certainly able to heal; and yet Timothy still used a little wine, Epaphroditus was also sick and not healed, and that Paul's eyes had gone so bad that he could not see small letters. But I also mentioned many in Scripture who had been healed. Whereupon brother Meek replied that the way I had answered was actually no answer at all. It was at this moment that I instantly realized what keeping the law was. Were the Bible to give us the statutes in successive steps, we could easily follow God's instruction. And such could be called the keeping of the law. But God wants us to have fellowship with Him directly and follow after the revelation He gives. Only then can the Holy Spirit work.

People like to have everything clearly defined in the Bible. For example, concerning the very matter of divine healing, we would like to see the Bible spell out plainly whether or not God will heal us. Yet in the Bible we have on the one hand sickness healed and on the other hand sickness unhealed. The Bible does not set forth a rule in this matter. For as in all matters God does not want His Church merely to keep the dead letter without coming before Him to ask. He takes pleasure in having us pray before Him and quietly wait. He does not want us to have any reliance upon anything except himself.

The law is the past wish of God, not His present desire. Men always try to learn God's present desire through His past wish. But God looks for us to commune with Him, and through the Holy Spirit come to know his present desire. He does not want us merely to keep the law. Hence, we need to have fresh communion with God every day in order to know His will.

The law has its second-hand effect in regulating one's life. But God has no desire to prearrange everyday church life. He wants to teach us how to maintain moment-by-moment communion with Him that we may know His will concerning ourselves. Were I to fix the life of a certain worker, he might be able to keep my rules for a day, a week, even a month without ever needing to have fellowship with me or ever needing to inquire of me about any matters. Such is the effect of the law. All who are able to do God's will without ever having fellowship with Him are but keeping the law.

81

In Shanghai, I had a servant. He was a brother in the Lord. One day I came to realize how it was indeed best for me to serve the Lord with my spirit and not by law, because that was what the Lord desired. I wanted to test this out by seeing if I could succeed in treating my servant with the spirit and not with the law. In ordinary circumstances it is generally convenient to follow the law that is set down. If I were to lay down laws and directives, my servant would find it easy to follow and I myself must also keep it. But I agreed with my servant that I would not give him any instruction beforehand, and that he must not decide for himself but come and ask me on each occasion before proceeding to do anything. Several times, while I was talking with a friend, he interrupted our conversation and asked if I wanted to eat or drink something. I told him to wait. As a result, my servant found it much easier to serve according to rules than to have to ask me each time. From this we can see that keeping the law is quite easy, but working according to the leading of the Holy Spirit is not so easy. Regardless whether easy or not easy, God's desire is clear. We cannot take the easy way. We must walk in God's ordained path, which is not to live under the law but to live under the Spirit.

Life in the Spirit

Life in the Spirit has no set rule. It lays aside all dead rules and seeks directly the will of God. It can be likened to the illustration of my servant cited above. After he has swept the floor, he does not know what the next work should be for him to do. Should he serve a meal at twelve o'clock or do something else? But life in the Spirit is very much like that: work only when there is the revelation of the Holy Spirit and at other times just wait on the Lord. Let us cite another example. How do we know whether a person is saved and ready for baptism? Should we examine him with every article of the truth on salvation and baptism? And if he can answer all the questions, can he then receive baptism? This would be doing things according to the law.

On the other hand, suppose you meet an old country lady who is illiterate and ignorant of Bible terminology. You question her about her regeneration, repentance, forgiveness and so forth. On none of these questions is she able to answer, yet she has peace in her heart. Will you allow her to be baptized? The issue does not lie in whether the candidate for baptism can pass your procedure and answer your various questions. It rests in whether she is really saved. Many country folk are not familiar with terminology, but they truly have the peace and the joy of the Lord within. Such people, though their minds be less bright than ours, are truly saved souls.

During meetings in Shanghai for the breaking of bread, strangers frequently visited us without previous notice. How long must we ask them to wait before they are allowed to partake of the bread and wine? Wait a week or a month according to some rule? If we know that the visitor is saved, can we not immediately invite him to partake of the bread and wine? There should be no need to wait.

Let us never lay down any law, but let the Holy Spirit work in each person. Everything in the Bible is living, that is to say, living in the Holy Spirit. If we turn all Biblical things into rules and regulations, they become dead. In order for Bible truth to be living, it must be in the Spirit. Take, for example, how on one occasion you received a message from the Lord, preached it, and many got saved. Next time you thought that because the last time you gave this same message it saved many souls it would certainly obtain the same result again. So you decide to preach the same message, but this time nobody got saved. You reflect that the message which saved souls before would no doubt save souls again. Nevertheless, it did not save any soul. Let us realize that the same message, if it is delivered in the Spirit, can and will indeed save souls; if repeated according to the law, however, it cannot save souls. Such is the difference between that which is done according to the Spirit and that which is done according to the law.

All that is not according to the living guidance of the Holy Spirit is the law. How frequently we use our past guidance of the Holy Spirit as today's guidance. Yet we need to learn that past guidance used today turns into a matter of the law. Do not imagine that since the Holy Spirit led once before, He will necessarily give the same leading today. Copying yesterday's leading is walking according to the law. Even in obeying Bible truth it can also become a matter of obeying the law. Today if you receive baptism only because the Bible says so, without also inwardly being led by the Spirit, this, too, can turn into a matter of observing the law. We must do what the Bible says, plus have an inner leading. The joining of these two gives accurate guidance.

Someone argues that because the Bible does not say a certain thing is wrong, therefore it must be right. This is altogether a thing of law. Many write and ask if to do or to say such and such a thing is wrong. My answer is: Do you have the Holy Spirit in you? If you do, why not learn to know the Spirit's guidance within you? I am not a fortune-teller, so I cannot know God's will for you. You instead must learn to recognize the inner guidance of the Holy Spirit.

In living according to the leading of the Holy Spirit, the first question we should ask ourselves is, What does the Holy Spirit say? Delay asking what the Bible says until a little later. Always first ask what our inside says. Today the majority of believers will first search to see what the Bible says; they do not first ask what the Holy Spirit in them says. This is rather abnormal. New Testament believers have the Holy Spirit indwelling them, which is a most precious reality. We ought to learn to know the leading of the Spirit within us. In the Bible can be found a distinction between principle and command. A believer needs indeed to keep the command of the Bible, but he must also practice the principle behind the command. For example, let us consider the subject of head-covering. If you practice head-covering simply because of 1 Corinthians 11, you are still as uncovered. For whoever keeps the word of the Bible without having the Spirit's leading in keeping the word is not acting any differently from that one who disobeys the word. Such keeping is a keeping of the letter and is in appearance only. The issue, therefore, is what does the Lord say within you? If it is indeed the Spirit of the Lord who leads you to obey a certain truth in the Bible, your action is truly an obedience to God.

The Old Testament period was the dispensation of the law. Today, though, is the New Testament era. Unfortunately the Church today has too many Judaized Christians. They take the Bible as the law and try to keep the law. Many simply ask others what they should do. This shows they are unable to seek after the Holy Spirit that is within them. All these actions are abnormal.

Guidance of the Spirit Confirmed by the Bible

Sheep know the voice of their shepherd. Many surmise that if they did not know the letters of the Bible they could not know the rules of holy living, and thus they would sin every day. In fact, however, the opposite is the truth. Depending on the guidance of the Holy Spirit is far better than depending on our own keeping of the Bible. For we may forget, but the Spirit of God never forgets. You will therefore probably ask, If the work of the Holy Spirit is so important, do we still need the Holy Bible? In theory, the guidance of the Spirit within us should be enough; but in practice, because our understanding of the inward guidance is subject to error, we still are in need of the Holy Bible. In other words, though we follow the inward guidance of the Holy Spirit and not just follow the teaching of the Holy Bible, yet we check our everyday inward guidance with the Bible. As we obey both the inward and the outward guidance, we are truly obeying God. Hence, we must have the guidance of the Spirit within and obey the teaching of the Bible without. We must always check our inward guidance with the Bible teaching. If it does not agree with the Bible, such guidance is not the leading of the Holy Spirit but is the working of our emotion. The root of all things lies within.

In Chefoo, two people one day asked me whether they should leave their denomination. I answered them that I did not know. They then said, "Does that mean that you oppose our leaving the denomination?" So I asked them this instead: "May I ask you, How is life in the denomination? Is your inner life while in the denomination overflowing? If so, you should remain in. Otherwise, you should come out." It is therefore not a matter of right or wrong, but an issue of life.

Also in Chefoo, a well-known lady missionary sought me three times to talk about sects. On the first two occasions I refused to talk with her. On the last occasion, due to her determination and also because of my being led by the Holy Spirit, I only used five minutes to talk with her. Then we had tea together. I simply told her I was in a big circle and that she was in a small circle within that big circle. Two days later she came early in the morning to see me and to tell me that on the previous night she had sent out three letters of resignation. I said to her, "You should not be influenced by me. This thing must only be done by God. God alone can tell you to leave a denomination." "Well", she replied, "last night as I sought God, I saw that the small circle within the big circle is a state chosen by men, and such a choice of man is sin. I felt it was God's will for me to leave the denomination. So last night I rose up and wrote those letters of resignation." I shook her hand. Thereafter, she walked positively in the way of the Lord, and was never negative.

We who do the work of the Lord should be careful to teach the believers to allow not only the Bible to lead them but the Holy Spirit to guide them inwardly as well. We must not use outward standards to unify the saints in order to maintain an external harmony. If so, the Holy Spirit will have no place and no outlet. We must not be a Moses giving people only the letters of the law. For our law is the Holy Spirit: "the law of the Spirit of life in Christ Jesus" (Rom. 8.2). The Holy Spirit teaches us all things: "the anointing [the teaching of the Holy Spirit] which ye received of him abideth in you, and ye need not that any one teach you; but as his anointing teacheth you concerning all things, and is true, and is no lie, and even as it taught you, abide ye in him" (1 John 2.27 mgn.). We must learn to hearken to the guidance of the Holy Spirit within us. By only keeping the outward law we just might end up living apart from God. But if we live by the inward Holy Spirit, we cannot for one moment depart from God and live.

8. The Function of the Anointing Oil[*]

Before God, Anointing Oil Is Sanctification

Leviticus 8 narrates how Aaron was anointed, and Leviticus also speaks of his subsequent ministry of offering sacrifices. Before David became King he too was first anointed with oil, by Samuel. Then he began to serve God according to the ministry God had given him (see 1 Sam. 16.12-13). All this clearly shows that ministry follows anointing. For a person to have a ministry before God, he must first have received an anointing. Even the Lord Jesus followed the same order: "The Spirit of the Lord is upon me, because he anointed me to preach good tidings to the poor: he hath sent me to proclaim release to the captives, and recovering of sight to the blind, to set at liberty them that are bruised, to proclaim the acceptable year of the Lord" (Luke 4.18-19). So in looking through God's word, we find that one who is useful in God's hand must first have received an anointing from Him. If he has not been anointed, he can neither serve God nor work for God.

This matter of having the anointing oil may quite easily be viewed as an outward thing in the minds of God's children. We may quickly link anointing oil with power, as Peter said (see Acts 10.38). It is true that anointing oil and power are associated together because God anointed Jesus of Nazareth with the Holy Spirit and power. Indeed, the Holy Spirit and power are linked together, and the Holy Spirit is the power of God. Nevertheless, even though the Holy Spirit as power in man is the result of anointing, it is not all that God has in mind when He anoints. We should understand that the primary significance of being anointed is not that we have been granted power to speak in tongues or to do wonders and miracles. Rather, it is the fact that we have been set apart for God.

---

[*] Notes of message given at Shanghai, sometime during 1938-42, a more exact date unobtainable.—Translator

The anointing oil is mentioned many times in the Old Testament, but there we do not find it being linked with power. In the Old Testament, anointing has but one meaning; which is, that it signifies that the anointed belongs to God. Just as we say that such and such a book is ours and we stamp our seal upon it, so God says that this or that person is His and anoints him with oil. Anointing oil is applied to indicate separation: it is also to indicate sanctification: in short, it means that the person receiving the oil is being set apart to be entirely for God or to be holy for God.

This being entirely the Lord's is the first condition of spiritual ministry. No one can have a ministry before God if he has not been sanctified unto Jehovah. In fact, only those who are set apart for Jehovah have any ministries. They alone can work for God. Whenever consecration ceases, work also stops. Whenever the "setting apart" changes, then ministry changes too.

When the Holy Spirit came upon the Lord Jesus, the first consequence was not for Him to commence working; rather, it was the receiving of God's recognition: "This is my beloved Son" (Matt. 3.17). This was the word spoken at that moment by God. Hence, anointing expresses God's right of possession. Here is a person about whom God can say, "He is Mine," about whom God can say, "He is to be sent and used by Me." Only then do we see that there is power. Yet it is only natural that there would be power. And the result is that the poor shall hear the gospel, the blind shall see, the captives shall be freed, and the acceptable year of the Lord shall be proclaimed.

Anointing Oil Is Power upon Others

God anointed Jesus of Nazareth with the Holy Spirit and with power. Then the Lord Jesus went about doing good and healing all who were oppressed of the devil. See again Acts 10.38. It says there that God anointed Him. What is this anointing? It is twofold: the Holy Spirit, and also power. This is both wonderful and precious. For the Holy Spirit upon us is the anointing oil, but upon others it is power. The power of the Spirit is discovered in others, but in you yourself it is the anointing oil. When the anointing is upon you, people touch power through you.

Consequently, our consecration before God naturally produces power upon others. So that the matter of power is not the first issue here, it is but the second. If the issue of consecration is solved before God, the issue of power on others is automatically resolved. Whenever consecration becomes a problem, power also becomes a problem. Anointing always gives power. This can be seen in David. This can also be seen in Aaron.

Anointing Oil Is Teaching in Us

As you learn to serve God, you often discover one particular fact, which is, that when you stand up to speak, you clearly have the anointing upon you if you truly speak for God. You do not have to force yourself or to exert great strength in speaking. You know indeed that you have the anointing upon you. Your words are quite common and simple, and yet the more you speak, the more powerful are your words. You sense the anointing. And when you sense the anointing, others feel the power. On the other hand, sometimes when you are speaking, you feel like a blown-out tire. You sense no life and people do not find power. The difference is in the anointing. Where there is anointing, there is power. But when there is no anointing, there will be no power. Hence, anointing upon you yourself means quickening; in others whom you touch it means power.

"And as for you, the anointing which ye received of him abideth in you, and ye need not that any one teach you; but as the anointing teacheth you concerning all things, and is true, and is no lie, and even as it taught you, abide ye in him" (1 John

2.27 mgn.). The word here is very comprehensive. The anointing shall teach us in all things. Divine teaching is vastly different from human teaching. Man's teaching is very complicated, for it involves many reasons and many words. But the teaching of the anointing is not so. It does not tell you many, many things, nor does it use many, many words. It teaches you quite simply by its presence or absence. This is its characteristic. Suppose, for example, you today are going to do a certain thing. If this is of the Lord, then when you make a move, you have the anointing; and thus you know that this is right. If, on the other hand, this is something you should not do, you will immediately feel like a tire blown out. Then you likewise know that this is wrong. The teaching of the anointing does not employ or involve reasoning. To the contrary, were reasoning involved, our human mind would have to be replaced since our mind, being so inferior to God's mind, has no way to understand His reason.

In view of all this, our sense of right and wrong must be judged according to the presence or absence of the anointing and not according to reason. All the children of God should learn a lesson here: in things pertaining to God we do not reason but look for a quickening sense from the Holy Spirit. Ofttimes as we attempt to do something, we can think of its reasonableness. But as we begin to do it, we feel as though we are accomplishing it alone since the Lord is not present with us. This indicates that there is no anointing. It also tells us we are wrong.

Take as another example your attempt to communicate to others. If you have no anointing, the more you talk the less the strength, and the longer you talk the emptier within. You sense an incredible dryness. On the other hand, if you have an anointing and a burden in you, the more you work the louder the amen inside you. You feel easy and light. You know this is what God wants you to say and do.

Therefore, no child of God should make any move if he does not sense the anointing in him. Were he to move on his own, he would instantly feel dead. Without the anointing, the more active he is outwardly, the more chilly he feels within, and others cannot touch anything. But with an anointing, others can feel there is power coming out of him. So, then, the consequence of this anointing for God's servant is teaching and knowledge; and for others it is power.

Many brethren are seeking for power and many are seeking for life. The word of God tells us, however, that "death worketh in us, but life in you" (2 Cor. 4.12). All who seek life in themselves shall never find life, since it is death that works in us in order for life to be in others. Similarly, let us not look at ourselves to see if we have power. Let us simply ask ourselves, Do we have the anointing oil? Anointing in us means power in others. If we seek for power, power may not come at all. And if it does come, it will most likely be only the external, miraculous and sensational kind of power, not that spiritual power spoken of in God's word.

How sad that some of God's children are seeking a power that can be felt! They think if they are conscious of power, they have the assurance of being useful to other people. This is altogether wrong. For what we need to pay attention to is not power, but anointing. Do we abide in the Lord in obedience to the teaching of the anointing? Anything which is not done in accordance with the teaching of the anointing will not give life to people. We may say many words which please itching ears. We may even say many meaningful words. But without the anointing we will immediately sense there is neither spiritual reality nor life. Only when we ourselves have the anointing before God will people naturally be helped, touch life, and even touch the Lord himself.

There is another point we must take note of here. The anointing of which we have been speaking is not just for the individual, nor is it for an individual alone to experience. It is for the body of Christ. The precious oil which had been poured upon Aaron's head ran down upon the beard and came all the way down upon the skirt of his garments (see Ps. 133.2). Under such situation, you realize how good and how pleasant it is (see v.1). Consequently, we not only seek the teaching of the anointing in us individually; we also seek for the teaching of the anointing throughout the body of Christ. Believers do not receive merely the guidance of the anointing that dwells within them individually, they also receive the guidance of the anointing that dwells in the body of Christ. For there in the Body, the Lord orders and leads in many things. How, then, can we go against the anointing in the Body?

We can illustrate it in this way. A certain brother was scheduled to lead a meeting, but he felt empty within. So he asked another brother to take his place. On the way, that brother felt he should give his testimony. Ordinarily he did not like to give a testimony, but this time he did because the anointing in him felt that way. It so happened that evening that two friends who had not come to the meeting for quite some time were present. They had quit coming previously because they had heard the gospel a number of times but had failed to understand anything. That evening they were urged to come again, and the brethren were praying for them, asking God to give a suitable word. The result was that the brother's testimony, as guided by the anointing, was given especially for these two friends. This is an example of the teaching of the anointing working both in us as individuals and in us as a corporate body. Let us always remember that we can never sense God more than the anointing upon us. The measure of the anointing in us is the limit of our service to God. Any excess will cause loss. We can only keep within the boundary the Lord has appointed to us.

After we truly experience the anointing, we begin to know what the ministry of the word of God is. We come to know how to serve Him with His word. For when we have the anointing, we have His word. Therefore, we serve God according to the anointing. It is God who causes us to notice what He notices. It is God who gives us word by which to serve Him and to serve His children.

Finally, I would exhort all you brothers and sisters here to consecrate yourselves thoroughly to God. All ministries are based on consecration. The anointing which God gives you proves you are His. With that anointing, you have the consciousness that you are His. You are the Lord's. With the anointing, you are aware of what the Lord wants you to do. And when you carry it out, there will be power upon other people. That power is not like the power we imagine in our mind which enables us to speak loudly in the pulpit or to perform wonders and miracles. No, this power enables people to touch life when you serve. This power is the result of none other than the divine anointing. May God bless us that we may abide in the Lord in accordance with the teaching of His anointing.

9. The Body Being Anointed*

The Bible shows us that God's anointing oil is for the one who fully satisfies His heart, even His Son Christ Jesus. Why, then, is the body of Christ, the Church, also anointed? Psalm 133 tells us that the precious oil which was poured upon Aaron's head ran down his beard and came down upon the skirt of his garments. When a person is anointed, the oil is poured upon the head, not upon the body of the anointed. But after the oil is poured upon his head, it flows down till it covers the entire body. This is a picture of Christ and the Church. The head is Christ, and the body is the Christ. Christ is the Anointed of God, and the Church is His body. So that when Christ is anointed, His entire body is also anointed. Christ is the great Anointed One, we the members are little anointed ones. Yet we are not anointed individually, but are anointed together in Christ at His anointing. We can never be anointed in ourselves. For the Scripture says, "Upon the flesh of man shall it [the holy anointing oil] not be poured" (Ex. 30.32a). We are therefore anointed in Christ.

Condition for Anointing Is the Natural Being Buried

Luke 3.22 speaks of what happened to the Lord after He was baptized in the river Jordan: "the Holy Spirit descended in a bodily form, as a dove, upon him, and a voice came out of heaven, Thou art my beloved Son; in thee I am well pleased." Again, in Luke 4.18, we read: "The Spirit of the Lord is upon me, because he anointed me to preach good tidings to the poor. . ." Hence after His baptism in the river Jordan, the Lord received the anointing of the Holy Spirit. Genesis 8 narrates how after the flood Noah opened the window of the ark and sent forth a dove. Inasmuch as the dove found no resting place for

---

* Notes of one of the messages given by the author at a conference held in Shanghai, August 1939.—Translator

the sole of her foot, she returned to the ark, for the waters were still on the face of the earth. (Noah's ark passing through the flood is a type of baptism.) At Christ's baptism, the Spirit of God descended upon Him as a dove. This indicates that He received the anointing of the Holy Spirit at the time of baptism. We too receive the anointing of the Spirit at our baptism.

Baptism signifies the burial of all the old and the natural. Anointing after baptism suggests that the flesh must be buried before we can receive the anointing of the Holy Spirit. If it were not because of the Lord we would not be able to come up out of the water because all which belongs to us ourselves is destined to be buried. That which can rise up after burial is on resurrection ground for it is in Christ. We are baptized in Christ; that is to say, in Him and with Him we pass through death and burial and we experience resurrection. So when He received the anointing, we too were anointed. In Him we died, were buried, resurrected, and anointed.

The Use of Anointing

What is the value of the anointing? Through the anointing, grace flows to the whole body of Christ. The usefulness of the anointing is in maintaining the relationship between the Body and the Head. It is also useful in affirming the relationship among the members of the Body. The anointing is the function of the Holy Spirit in men.

The relationship of the Holy Spirit with Christ and the Church can be likened to the nerve system found in the human body. This system connects and directs all the various parts of the body. Through the nerve system the head controls the action of all its members. It is also through the nerve system that all the members are joined with one another. All the members of the body function in obedience to the direction of the nerve system. In following the nerve system, they follow the head. In like manner, in the spiritual body it is the Holy Spirit who communicates the thought of the Head to all its members. As members of the body of Christ we must submit ourselves to the authority of the Holy Spirit. Our submission is submission to the Head. When we grieve the Holy Spirit, we thwart the relationship between ourselves and the Head. How do we hold fast the Head? Through obeying the Holy Spirit.

The Teaching of the Anointing

In the Bible the Holy Spirit is symbolized by many different things, such as wind, living water, fire, and so forth. All these show forth the various aspects of the work of the Holy Spirit. But what is presented in 1 John 2.27 is especially precious. Here it speaks of the anointing of the Holy Spirit which is the teaching of the Holy Spirit. How does the Spirit teach? He teaches by the anointing. How do we come to know the will of God? Not by research, nor by balancing pro and con, but by the teaching of the anointing. It is the Holy Spirit who communicates the mind of Christ to us. We have no need to ask all the time, "Is this the will of God?" For "we have the mind of Christ" (1 Cor. 2.16b). When the Head wants a certain member of the Body to move, He makes him know this by the Holy Spirit. As we obey the anointing, life will freely flow in us. But if we resist the anointing our relationship with the Head is disrupted and the flow of life also ceases.

Why is it that many believers do not know the Lord's guidance? It is because they are not in subjection to the Head. For the anointing does not come up from the Body; rather, it comes down from the Head. Only when believers are directly under the Head can they receive the anointing that runs from the Head to the whole Body.

The anointing may also be referred to as "the anointing of the Lord." We know that oil is a substance which is soft and soothing in its application. The Holy Spirit does not teach us in any rough or wild way. For here He is not likened, as elsewhere in the Bible, to the blowing of strong wind or to the burning of fire. On the contrary, here He is likened to a soothing ointment that is applied within us. Such is the way the Holy Spirit instructs us. Where the anointing is, there is God's work. For God's work depends not on words, Bible interpretation, reasons or judgments. God works within us. His inner guidance comes as a kind of inner life-consciousness. This kind of life-consciousness is the anointing of the Holy Spirit. The Lord does not employ external forces to control the body. Rather, we are told that "the life was the light of men" (John 1.4).

The way to know God's will is not by inquiring if this or that matter is right or wrong, but by sensing whether you have life or not. If you sense death in yourself in a matter, it discloses the fact that there is no positive anointing. And if you proceed to do it without such anointing, then you are not moving under the authority of the Lord. Sometimes as you go visiting those in need, for example, you sense a freezing within you. Yet according to the Biblical principle as well as human concern and compassion, you should go. But the further you go, the colder your heart becomes. This indicates that the Holy Spirit is instructing you not to proceed. On the other hand, at other times when you go visiting, you are as one anointed with precious ointment, you feeling quite natural and comfortable in proceeding. This too is the anointing of the Holy Spirit in you, which in this case produces the teaching for you to go. If at that time you follow this anointing, your strength increases and amens will be multiplied in you.

The essence of the teaching of the anointing of the Holy Spirit is not a matter of right or wrong, good or evil, yea or nay. It is essentially an inner consciousness of life. The works of many people are done according to the way of the tree of the knowledge of good and evil, its fruit having originally been eaten by the very first man. This is the so-called principle of right and wrong that had its beginning in Adam. But in Christ, God's working is an issue of life, a matter of the anointing of the Holy Spirit. Where the anointing is, there is life. The presence of the anointing and life justifies the matter and confirms it as being of God.

As a consequence, people who are intelligent and knowledgeable in Bible truth may not necessarily understand God's will and work better. Sometimes brothers and sisters in the rural areas know far more of the will and workings of God, for what they depend on is not knowledge but life. If the ability to know the divine will and work were solely a matter of reason and intelligence, then God would be guilty of partiality and unfairness, and woe to the illiterate country folk who have not the intelligence to know God's will! But God is not partial to anyone. Whether you are intelligent or not, clever or foolish, the teaching of the anointing of the Holy Spirit is in you. If you follow the Spirit's anointing within you, you will know God's will and do His work.

The Anointing and the Law

In the Old Testament period, when people brought out God's word, it became the law to them. In the New Testament era, if people bring out God's word without at the same time having the anointing of the Holy Spirit, God's word too becomes law. Let us notice, however, that whenever the Lord Jesus brought forth God's word, that word became life and spirit (see John 6.63b). The apostles also brought forth God's word as life and spirit. On the other hand, the Pharisees, although they too brought forth God's word, did not have the anointing of the Holy Spirit. So their words became dead law to be rigorously kept.

Many believers receive baptism and the laying on of hands according to the word in the Bible, yet to them these words are nothing but laws to be kept. Whoever follows only the letter of the word, that one is a disciple of Moses and not a disciple of Christ. Christians who walk rightly are those who have the anointing of the Lord. In the body of Christ there is no law save "the law of the Spirit of life in Christ Jesus" (Rom. 8.2): that is, the anointing of the Holy Spirit. Hence we who live in the body of Christ must live by the Spirit's anointing and not by the letter of the law. We must do everything according to the anointing of the Holy Spirit—which is to say, according to the teaching of the Holy Spirit.

How to Be Anointed

How can we be anointed? Psalm 133 is a principal passage in the Old Testament on anointing. We know that Psalms 120 to 134 are together referred to as "the songs of degrees or ascents." These were the songs sung by the children of Israel as they gathered together three times a year to appear before the Lord in Jerusalem and ascend Mount Zion—God's habitation. These fifteen songs—whose subject matter, though varied, are all interrelated—served as the singing repertoire of the Israelites as they, in keeping with the progressive degree of meaning of the songs themselves, ascended step by step and higher and higher towards their goal.[*] Needless to say, moreover, during their pilgrimage, they left off speaking about economics, education, war, politics or any other mundane topic. Instead, as they traveled along, their hearts were turned more and more towards Zion, towards God himself; and so from all over the land they ascended towards Jerusalem degree by degree in keeping with the content and character as it were of each song of ascent. And when these pilgrims arrived at the place and moment for singing the next to the last of these songs, they broke forth with the opening words of Psalm 133: "Behold, how good and how pleasant it is for brethren to dwell together

---

[*] For an in-depth study of these fifteen Psalms, the reader may wish to consult Stephen Kaung, The Songs of Degrees (New York: Christian Fellowship Publishers, 1970).—Translator

in unity! It is like the precious oil upon the head, that ran down upon the beard, even Aaron's beard; that came down upon the skirt of his garments" (vv.1-2).

Now this dwelling together by these Israelites, which was the near-culmination of their pilgrimage begun weeks and months before, resulted in a corporate unity that was devoid of division and independence. There on Mount Zion in the presence of God they put aside all former disagreement, jealousy, hatred and so forth. And just as is described in the verses of this psalm, these gathered united Israelites were able to receive God's anointing: even God's blessing of life forevermore (see v.3). They experienced the spiritual reality of what is pictured for us in physical terms by the psalmist: for as the oil is poured upon the head of Aaron the high priest, it flows down upon and beyond the beard and even reaches to the very skirt of his garments, thus making it possible for everything that is beneath Aaron's head to be touched by the anointing oil too.

Psalm 133 in the Old Testament is comparable to much of Ephesians 4 in the New Testament, especially with respect to the twin matters of unity and fellowship. When we who are in the body of Christ diligently keep the unity of the Holy Spirit (see Eph. 4.3), we have His anointing. We need to stand under the Head—even Christ our Great High Priest—and live in His body in order to have the anointing. Many fail to receive guidance because they have not stood in the proper place. They have not stood under the Head; they have not obeyed the anointing of the Head; they have not even lived as it were in the Body. For us to be anointed and to enjoy true Christian fellowship, we must submit ourselves under the headship of Christ on the one side and live in the Body on the other.

The *basis* of the believer's fellowship is grounded in Christ. We can fellowship with one another because Christ is the life of the Body and Christ is the Head. On the other hand, the enjoyment of fellowship is grounded in the Holy Spirit. The more we enjoy the anointing of the Spirit the more we are in the fellowship of the Body. Whether or not we believers enjoy fellowship, however, is something conditional; it depends on whether our natural life is being dealt with; that is to say, we must let the cross deal deeply with the flesh and natural life. Our natural flesh is worthy of death, worthy of being crucified on the cross and laid in dust and ashes. We cannot rely on our own mind: we are not fit to follow our own will: we must give Christ absolute sovereignty and let Him be Lord. By accepting the dealing of the cross over our natural life, obeying the headship of Christ, and living out the Body life, we shall have the anointing of the Holy Spirit and shall enjoy the fellowship of the Body.

PART THREE

SPIRITUAL JUDGMENT (OR DISCERNMENT)*

---

* Part Three consists of four messages that cover this overall subject. They were presented in Chinese by the author before an audience of his fellow-workers on four consecutive days in 1948: 29 and 30 September and 1 and 2 October. As was the case with the messages that comprise Part One of this volume, the author delivered these messages on spiritual judgment during the lengthy First Workers Training Session that was convened during the summer of 1948 at the Conference Center which had been established by the author on Mount Kuling, near Foochow, China. Derived from the extensive notes taken down in Chinese by several participants present at the Workers Conference, the contents of these four messages have now been translated into English.—Translator

1. The Principles of Spiritual Judgment

The judgment we shall be talking about here is not the judgment of a court as seen in modern society. It is spiritual judgment. First and foremost, we must recognize that unless we can discern, we will have trouble in serving the Lord. For we can be too easily deceived. On this matter of judgment or discernment, therefore, we need to take note of a few principles.

The Five Principles (Criteria) of Judgment

The first principle concerns truth or the discipline of the Holy Spirit. As you converse with a brother or a sister, you should notice if his or her lessons are learned from the truth or from the discipline of the Holy Spirit. Some incline to the one side and some lean to the other. Some bend to the truth, while some tilt to the discipline of the Spirit. Learning from truth means that a person acts according to the word and relevant teaching of the Bible which he has heard. Or he obeys the Lord when he is moved by what he reads of the Scriptures or what he hears from preaching. On the other hand, learning from the discipline of the Holy Spirit means that after a person has experienced the dealing hand of the Lord upon him, he is gradually broken by the Lord and is delivered from his early stage of insubordination, murmuring, fret, or opinions into a state of obedience. This is a learning from the circumstances of his environment as so arranged by the Holy Spirit.

Hence one person may learn to obey through teaching and another person may learn to obey through dealings. As a worker for the Lord you need to discern on which side of this issue that brother or sister belongs. If there is learning on both sides, that is the best. With such a balance as this, a Christian can walk uprightly. God's worker must therefore be acquainted with both ways of learning. Then he can detect which way is absent or present in a given brother or sister. He must know in his heart where the need is in this person or that. Some believers know nothing about the discipline of the Holy Spirit, and hence they are hard and raw. Others are in just the opposite ignorance; that is, they have no ability to learn from truth and relevant teaching. Thus they are ignorant of many truths and are not obedient to many commandments in the Bible.

The second principle or criterion by which to render judgment has to do with the outside versus the inside. Some have only the first and none of the second. They may learn much in matters of the truth, but their obedience to these truths is all outward: they are outwardly baptized, they outwardly practice head-covering, and so forth. Nevertheless, there is no inward learning. Some others, though, may encounter various unpleasant situations and pass through many difficulties—all these being the result of the discipline of the Holy Spirit upon their lives—and yet all these things touch only the outside, stop there and never reach the inside. From this we may conclude that a life under the discipline of the Holy Spirit may be lived outwardly or lived inwardly.

Let us take, for example, the case of a person who is sick. He is one who is under the Spirit's discipline. Now on the one hand he may appear to be submissive outwardly, but on the other hand he does not have inward joy and praise because of his illness. Though outwardly he may declare, "If I am sick, I am sick," this is at most patiently and passively accepting the discipline; it is not an inward attitude of praise and thanksgiving. Such discipline has merely touched the outside. Yet if in accepting the sickness he not only patiently endures the discipline of the Holy Spirit but also takes the further step of praising the Lord, such discipline impacts upon the person inwardly.

As we have seen, however, this person can neither give thanks nor praise. He is simply forcing himself to subject himself under the mighty hand of God. The impact of such discipline upon him is only outward. But if he can bring himself to praise and thank God for giving him this discipline and if his heart can be full of joy, then God's discipline will reach its end in that life. When discipline becomes something inward, the person will not ask for quick relief from his sickness so as to feel comfortable. Instead, he will be able to praise and thank the Lord for what He has done and to confess that what the Lord has done is all well.

As another example, someone may see the error of being in a sect and come out of it; but in his having done so, sectarianism has unfortunately not left him. For his love of the brethren has not increased and his fellowship is still restricted. For instance, when he meets a brother he may appear to be open, even embracing and kissing that brother. Even so, though he exhibits an outward expression of brotherly love, there is no real sense of love inwardly. All is acting and pretending. All is outward, not inward.

Let us who seek to serve the Lord understand that all the virtues mentioned in the Bible point to the being of a person, not his doing. So that in the process of discerning, we need to have a clear picture of the life of a given brother or sister as to whether it is inward or just outward. If only the latter, we must lead him to the inward. Many say a certain brother is very good. But how good is he? Is it an inward or an outward goodness? The difference is great. We must learn to distinguish the inward and the outward of a life.

The third principle or criterion to be used by God's workers in rendering judgment or discernment pertains to the issue of the spirit versus the mind. On the one hand many spiritual things register in man's spirit and on the other hand in man's mind. It is very difficult for some to judge from the words and terms which another person uses whether the thing to be judged is emanating from the spirit or from the mind. For people can adopt the same words and terms from either source because they have had little or no dealings of renewal in their mind. But if you as one who must judge in such matters have had spiritual experiences and have learned much in your spirit, then you can perceive whether a person's speech is coming from his mind or from his spirit. You can discern the inward difference. When someone speaks out of his spirit, you can touch that spirit as soon as he speaks. Conversely, you touch the mind of the speaker when he speaks out of his mind. Spiritual things that stay only in the mind become ideals which carry no spiritual value. Furthermore, if someone's spiritual life relies solely on mental knowledge, his life becomes empty and devoid of any spiritual worth. The lives of believers must not be managed by the mind.

Let us see, then, that to judge a speech whether it emanates from the spirit or from the mind is the initial step in spiritual discernment. He who cannot distinguish spirit from mind is unable to render spiritual judgment. Such an inability is a serious problem in divine service. For wherever we who serve the Lord come and go we must learn to discern. We must be able to sense at once whether a person's spirit or mind has come forth. For though the words may be the same, those which come out of the mind do not have the same flavor as the words which come out of the spirit. In Shanghai, people frequently reported that a certain brother spoke well. When I went to hear him, however, I found that all he said came out of his mind. I made the same discovery when another person was reported to have preached exceedingly well. In several contacts I then had with this man I could only meet his mind.

Let it be recognized that some words we hear spoken are from the spirit and some words from the mind; which means we must not be deceived by the spoken words. Sometimes young people may think they can speak the same words that other brothers have spoken, and even speak better. But actually those other brothers speak out of their spirit whereas the young people too often speak out of their mind.

The quality between the two is quite different. Yet unless you are able to discern this qualitative difference, you will be easily deceived. A person who grapples with God's word in his mind without any engagement of his spirit in the learning process may have something to say; but because his spirit was given no place, what he said was useless. A worker for the Lord must learn to differentiate between what is of the mind and of the spirit.

The fourth principle or criterion to follow when rendering spiritual judgment relates to the natural and the spiritual. When you who are God's worker are dealing with a brother or listening to his testimony, you should use your spirit to search out his spiritual condition. You might make up a list showing what kind of person he is naturally and what kind he is spiritually. As he opens his mouth, you will recognize what kind of man he is: whether clever, fast-speaking, lazy, confused, quick-tempered, careless, humorous, joking, talkative, naughty, inaccurate, or whatever. Each person has his own characteristics, and if you have the time, you can put the predominant characteristics of each person on a list, for no one is able to conceal himself for too long. True, at the beginning he may be able to control himself; eventually, though, he will expose himself, for as he continues to speak, he will reveal his characteristics to you. Hence when you listen, you can generally disregard his initial words since usually they are spoken under control. But after a while, his own self will begin to show forth, for "out of the abundance of the heart the mouth speaketh" (Matt. 12.34).

Now once you have discovered his natural characteristics, you can then shift your attention to the other facet to this to learn how he is before the Lord. Perhaps his temper has been dealt with; perhaps his speech or attitude or self-love has been dealt with. Through his experiences a person may have learned some lesson about physical problems. By this you may know that God has done something in his life. From the word of his testimony you can discern how much he has learned before the Lord, how much God has worked in his life, and how much Christ is being incorporated in him. All these are building up his life.

For this reason, you need to know a person both on the natural side and the spiritual side. You must determine what kind of a man he is naturally, and also how much upbuilding is taking place in his life. You should also take note how his spirit and natural characteristic blend together. With regard to some people, of course, this point may be rather hard to ascertain. Yet even if you are able to judge this, you may not be able to prescribe the remedy. For example, some people are quick in thought, but due to their much discipline, you will need to ask yourself whether such quickness needs to be dealt with. This depends on discerning whether their natural characteristic of quickness interferes with their being good Christians. How we must learn to discern! We need to know people's condition clearly before we can direct their way.

The fifth and final principle or criterion that needs to be mentioned has to do with distinguishing between the spirit and emotion: between what is emanating from a believer's spirit and what is emanating from his emotion. It is much easier to apprehend the difference between the spirit and the mind than to discern the difference between the spirit and emotion. It is quite difficult to differentiate when man's spirit comes forth and when his emotion comes forth. Even so, we still must learn this difference, for some speak out of their spirit while others speak out of their feelings.

The spirit, like the soul, has its knowledge and emotion. Spiritual knowledge differs from mental knowledge in that the latter proceeds from the mind and therefore you cannot touch the spirit at all. If a person's knowledge springs forth from his spirit you will inwardly sense reality and respond with an amen. You will feel comfortable inside. If a person's speech originates from his mind, though, his words may sound correct and yet you inwardly detest them.

Now when a believer's speech sallies forth from his spirit, it gives you a comfortable and joyful feeling. As his spirit comes forth, your spirit echoes. If, however, what he says arises from his emotion, it is difficult for you to discern whether he speaks from his emotion or from his spirit. If the spirit of a believer launches out with thought we will only sense his spirit and not his thought. But if his spirit pushes forth with emotion we can feel both, for the spirit is in the emotion. We will sense the spirit as well as the emotion. How easily we mistake emotion for spirit.

How, then, are we going to distinguish between these two? It is really difficult to explain, but I will try my best to elucidate. We say that when a person's spirit comes forth it carries with it emotion. If his emotion and spirit are at one, his spirit will be echoed in you. By this you know that his spirit is clean and gentle, yet strong. But when a person's spirit comes out with his emotion and you sense that his spirit and emotion do not agree, then his emotion is released but you cannot find his spirit. And as your spirit is being touched by his emotion you have a sense of being defiled. As a matter of fact, whenever there is emotion but not spirit present, you always feel inwardly polluted. When the spirit and emotion are one, however, you inwardly experience joy and can amen it. Now should we ever detect any defilement of our spirit, we must reject it altogether. In this entire matter, we must apply ourselves diligently to learn to discern between the spirit and emotion.

Basic Condition for Spiritual Judgment

Let me mention one more thing. In our endeavor to exercise spiritual judgment, there is a fundamental condition to be met: we ourselves must receive strict judgment before God. I cannot give you any method as to how to discern. I can only say that your knowledge of others depends on your knowledge of yourself. Unless you know yourself, you will not be able to know others. After you yourself have been strictly judged by God, you can easily discern your brothers and sisters. When another person's spirit comes forth, how can you know if his spirit is right or wrong? You can only know because you have inwardly learned your own lessons, you have passed through judgment, you have had inner experience. You can measure those things which come out from other people by your own experiences, and thus you will be enabled to know immediately where they stand. If there is a lesson you have not learned, then you cannot detect its error in others and thus you will unknowingly let it pass. But if in that area you have been severely dealt with by God, then as soon as something similar appears in others, you will know and recognize it at once.

Hence the basis of our knowledge of people is found in ourselves being judged. To the degree that we know ourselves, to that degree will we know our brothers and sisters. If we have not been judged before God, no amount of methods will be effective. What we ourselves have not passed through can never help other people through. But with sufficient dealing we shall be able to detect others' problems and help them get through their difficulties.

We ourselves need to have more dealing. The more we learn before God about ourselves the better we are able to know our brothers and sisters. Otherwise, we are unaware where and how they have gone wrong. We need to be dealt with by the Holy Spirit in large and small matters. What we ourselves have experienced enables us to understand the actions or proclivities of others. For as a matter of fact, men are more or less alike. Their temper, nature, desires and so forth are not that far apart. Their ways of error and sin lie within a limited range. Everyone is a descendant of Adam; all therefore inherit Adam's life. And hence, should we be enlightened to better know ourselves, it is almost certain that we can better know our entire world. Just bear in mind that in every descendant of Adam can be found a full-fledged Adam. It therefore becomes relatively easy to diagnose others if we have learned to know ourselves. Let us not fancy that if we can just learn a certain technique we can know people. No, we must first learn the lessons about ourselves before we can ever use any method. Our usefulness depends upon our willingness to be dealt with by God. Whatever dealings we avoid experiencing before God will be precisely those areas in which we cannot help others. So let us not be so foolish as to play truant in this regard. For if we do play truant, it will only lessen our spiritual usefulness.

What is ministry? Ministry is supplying others with what we have learned before God. No learning, no supply. All our happenings, arrangements and disciplines are for the sake of preparing us for the ministry. True discipline of the Holy Spirit increases the richness of ministry. The less you pass through, the less help you can give to others. The more difficulties you encounter and the more discipline you experience, the better you are able to lead people to fullness. The scope of ministry will be determined by the amount of the Spirit's discipline in your life. If you have not learned anything, then all you can say to your brothers and sisters are but trivial, humorous words— words which can never hit the target. But if you have learned much, you can discern whether or not people's problems have been resolved. Moreover, you will not be easily deceived.

Take, for example, the matter of the gospel. This is at least one issue about which you know something. No person can deceive or cheat you about whether or not he is saved. Even so, the principle will be the same for you when it comes to deeper spiritual issues: it all depends upon your learning and experience before the Lord. The more you learn, the sharper will be your discernment. A casual touch with a brother will quickly tell you what is wrong.

May I therefore beg you, for the sake of fulfilling your ministry in serving the Lord, that you gladly and willingly put yourself in God's hand and accept the discipline of the Holy Spirit. Unless there is a building up within, there can be no work without. All God's works are done deep within a man, not merely in his mind. Not because of two or three years' study of the Bible are you able to be a preacher. How easy it would be if the Lord merely required His disciples to recite some sermons. Instead, He desires to bring them through much practical learning.

The reason why we desire to know people is for the sake of helping them, not for the sake of curiosity. It is to build them up, not to destroy them. In order to be useful, we must unconditionally, unreservedly, and joyfully commit ourselves into God's hand and accept the discipline of His Holy Spirit. The measure of your acceptance here determines your future usefulness elsewhere. The more the discipline, the more the enlargement and usefulness. We should not instruct people merely with teaching. We must accept the discipline of the Holy Spirit that can lead us into spiritual fullness and service.

2. Spiritual Judgment: Using Our Spirit

Yesterday we spoke on the importance of spiritual judgment or discernment. Today we would talk more specifically about the importance of using our spiritual senses. Whenever you are communicating with people, you give them opportunity to talk so that you may have the opportunity to know and discern with your spirit. It is rather difficult to know a person if he keeps his mouth shut. It is rare that you are able to see through a silent man. You may perhaps sense the quality of his spirit, but you cannot explain it with understanding. Sometimes you may indeed detect something wrong with his spirit, but in what way it is wrong you cannot tell. In our messages about the character of God's workman, we mentioned how a worker needs to learn to listen.* He should cultivate the habit of listening. Even if a person is talking about nonsense or is just pretending, you still have to listen. Without having this habit of listening, you close the door to knowing people. For it is through people's speech that you come to know them. What is most to be feared is if they should keep their mouths shut. But once they talk, it becomes God's opportunity for us to get to know them. Especially with those talkative people, in fact, you are able to know them quite much.

When a person begins to talk, you should prepare your spirit to touch his spirit. Yesterday we mentioned five principles or criteria to follow in rendering judgment. With these five as a foundation, let us use our spirit to sense and to discern. For a person's spirit is manifested in his talking. He is not able for

---

* This particular trait—"able to listen"—is in fact the subject of the very first in a series of messages on the overall topic of "The Character of God's Workman" which the author delivered at this same lengthy summer workers conference on Kuling Mountain in 1948 at which the present messages on spiritual judgment were also given. See Watchman Nee, The Character of God's Workman (New York: Christian Fellowship Publishers, 1988), translated from the Chinese.—Translator

long to cover his spirit with words. For as he speaks, his spirit will come forth. While he is talking let us listen on the one hand and use our spirit to contact him on the other. It is certain that how he talks will disclose his spirit, and how a man's spirit is, reflects upon his person. Hence, when another person begins to speak, your spirit should be open, tender and ready for any impression to be registered in you. As we listen and use our spirit to touch another's spirit, we need to notice several conditions. These we shall now take up one by one and discuss.

Man's Seven Conditions

1. The spirit in a person: right or wrong?

As we listen and touch the spirit of a man, we must first of all detect whether his spirit is right or wrong. If your own spirit is open, you will discern within yourself whether that other man's spirit is right or wrong by the impression he leaves with you. Someone may say the right word, but his intention is wrong. Someone may fill his words with love, yet his spirit is hateful. Someone may utter gentle words, but soon thereafter he reveals a hard spirit. Though it is possible for intent and word to differ, nevertheless, inwardly his spirit follows out after his word.

Recall what the Lord once declared, that "out of the abundance of the heart the mouth speaketh" (Matt. 12.34b). Man's speech cannot be controlled by his will to such a degree that his spirit will never be disclosed. In the end he shall reveal himself through his own speech. In other words, his mouth cannot totally check his spirit. Sooner or later his accent will expose him. If, for example, a Galilean keeps his mouth shut, nobody can tell he is a Galilean. Once he opens his mouth, though, he is recognized as a Galilean by his very speech (see Mark 14.66-70).

Because the intent of someone may be triggered by pride, jealousy or boastfulness, his spirit will for sure be most wrong. As a consequence, we cannot simply hearken to his word; we must also try to detect his spirit. Let us not believe the word that is restrained by a person's will, for it cannot represent either the truth or himself; his spirit alone represents him. This is basic. A person's real condition is his spirit's condition, not his will-managed word. Many are deceived because they are unable to distinguish between word and spirit. In spite of what man may disclose his intention to be, let us take note of his spirit. The words of Absalom, for example, were quite right, but his spirit was quite wrong because his was a rebellious spirit. Hence we must always touch people's spirit. Then we shall truly know them and discern whose words are trustworthy.

2. Where man's strength is.

When a person commences to speak, his spirit, right or wrong, will soon come forth. As his spirit emerges, his inner condition is revealed. In listening to a person, attempt to find out where his strongest point is. Ask yourself what impression he has given you. Ferret out which part of that man is the strongest. If your spirit is open and tender before God, it will sense where his strength truly lies. As his strength is revealed, he makes a deep impression in you. He may be a subjective person or a stubborn person, and so as he speaks he will let his strong point be exposed. And in so doing, he will leave a distinct impression in you. A gentle person, as cited in James 3.17, is easy to be entreated. But with someone else you may beg for half a day and still not easily get an answer. A person who is subjective and strong-willed is difficult to be entreated. Someone may be a strongly emotional person who can easily be swayed. He may say words of love, but it may not be genuine love. If your spirit is clean and gentle you can quite easily touch a person's strong point, which more often than not will turn out to be his fundamental problem; and as such it is where he needs to be dealt with. We must therefore use our spirit to touch people's predominant characteristic and so come to know what kind of person we are dealing with.

3. Whether the spirit is closed.

Usually when you converse with a brother, you can touch his spirit. But sometimes man's spirit does not come forth. Even after holding conversation for quite a long while, you still are unable to touch his spirit. His real person is in hiding, where you cannot apprehend him. His real self is concealed so well that you just cannot figure him out. Such a person must have a serious defect, since God's people should be easy to contact: they live, or should be living, according to "the principle of amen." That is, whenever they act or speak, it causes the spirit in others to respond with an amen. Such should be the "natural" state of a Christian. Nevertheless, there are some people who always seem to be hidden or are shut within themselves, and so much so that others cannot say much. These are hidden ones. Nobody knows them, nor do they fellowship with anyone. This constitutes a very serious situation. Their isolating individualism is so strong that no one may touch their real person. They are thus severed from the fellowship of the Body.

True, a Christian should be deep, yet he must also disclose his real state and allow people to touch his spirit. He who forbids his spirit to be touched has cut himself off from fellowship. He has not learned any lesson of the Body and knows nothing of what fellowship is. Someone may have been a Christian for eight or ten years, and yet you could never touch his spirit through his speech. Such is a closed spirit. We must try to touch that person's inner man, for the spirit of him who is beyond touch constitutes a big problem in the Church. It is deemed in the world that the more unfathomable you are the better. This is not to be so with Christians. The spirit of a Christian needs to be open so that he can fellowship with others.

4. Is the person abnormal?

As you listen to a person talking, his word will show whether his emotion is strong, his mind the dominant characteristic, or that he is very subjective. Although such a person may be particularly strong in some area, he is nonetheless a normal person. However, there are people with a strong mind or a rich emotion who are so aggressive that they become what can only be termed abnormal. The thought of such a person is crooked. He is abnormal, strange, extreme. Indeed, he is a devious person. His psychological constitution differs from that of ordinary people. Yet such people are not that rare to find. Among a hundred people, there will always be a few abnormal ones. Their thought and action are quite different from that of ordinary folk. They will always be against others.

Now their problem is so great that the ordinary way of contacting them will be of no avail in helping them. They need a special way of being dealt with. As a matter of fact, they must be dealt with very strictly because their constitution is so devious. If the ordinary way is used, you may exhort such a person twenty times and each time you will be disappointed, for his character has already become so deeply set and entrenched in him. Hence you must have your eyes especially wide open to judge if he is such a devious person indeed.

5. Is there any pretension?

In discerning, you need to discover if that person is pretentious. A sanctimonious person can hardly make any progress before God for it appears he needs to be doubly dealt with by God. In an ordinary person, there is only the corrupted flesh present. But a hypocritical person adds a shell of falsehood to the corruption of his flesh. Now an ordinary person need only have his flesh dealt with. But a pretentious person must have not only his flesh dealt with; there must also be a dealing with that shell of falsehood he has: such as a false goodness, feigned piety, assumed humility, manufactured gestures, a make-believe mannerism, and so forth. For people like this to be delivered, a double effort is required. God must first destroy their falsehood, expose all their pretensions, demolish their unnaturalness, wreck all that appears more than they really are; and finally, He must deal drastically with their flesh.

As soon as you are in contact with a brother, you should learn whether he is transparent or pretending. If there is only outward appearance, he needs to be dealt with by God. You must ferret out the man's hypocrisy. The person who laughs before you today may be putting on a facade. He may not be really joyful. Or another person may speak good words and assume a fine manner, but after conversing with him for a while the experienced in the Lord's ways of dealing can sense he is not altogether right.

All who wish to be true servants of God need first to recognize falsehood in themselves. Some are deceived by others because they have become pretentious and dishonest themselves. In order to deal with other people, the would-be worker of God must first learn to judge all falsehood in his own self. All that is fabrication without inward initiation must be purified out. Only after he has dealt with his own falsehood can his spirit become quite clean and sensitive. He can then detect falsehood in others as soon as he encounters it. For his spirit will now react to all falsehood with discomfort, even anger, because it defiles him.

6. The condition of the person's spirit.

As your spirit touches people, the more scrupulous the touch the better. You must discover the condition of their spirit. The spirit of some seems to be timid; it withdraws as soon as it comes forth. If your spirit is clean, you can touch this timid spirit. You will encourage him a little in your talk with him. Or perhaps the spirit of someone has been wounded. This may be the case because in former days he may have had a family problem or he may have been misunderstood or ill-treated. When you find out about such a condition, you must seek how to help him. You may need as it were to pour wine and oil upon him. He should be assured of what you are doing. With someone else, however, you may need to "strike" him and intensify his wound in order for your assistance to be of any profit to him. On the other hand, there may be someone else who would be completely crushed if he were hurt or wounded further. But then again, another person's so-called wound may be only superficial, requiring you in this case to "strike" again. In dealing with people, you yourself must have the conviction as to whom wine and oil should be applied and upon whom deeper wounds need to be inflicted. In the case of some, you should comfort with the word of the Lord. In the case of others, you need to reprove with severe words. And in the case of still others, you must awaken their slumbering spirit. First find out his actual condition; then decide what treatment, whether light or heavy, to use. The spirit of some is in slumber; the spirit of others appears to be under heavy pressure. Some seem to be crushed; others appear to be unconcerned. Each condition is different.

To sum up, then, before you can deal with people, you need to learn the condition and cause of their spirit's situation. You must be clear about the one with whom you deal: you should not be vague. A worker must be so objective as to be able to discern man's spirit. A worker who uses his mind and mental knowledge to help people produces no spiritual value. What is the use of parroting some form of words? In short, God's worker must himself be dealt with in order to deal with and give help to others.

7. A kind of unknown spirit exists.

In dealing with people you will come to see that the six kinds of condition mentioned above relative to their spirit are comparatively common. Yet beyond these six conditions, there exists another kind. This is the unknown spirit, which is hard to decipher. As you listen to a person talk or give testimony, you sense he is not well, yet you cannot tell where his spiritual illness lies. The state of his spirit does not seem to fit any of the above six kinds of condition. You cannot pinpoint his problem. You sense there is something wrong, but only vaguely. Such a condition is usually the result of some unknown sin, most likely of some hidden sin; or else the result of something far more serious than sin, it perhaps being the result of even the work or attack of the devil. It may be due to some unexplained sin that gives Satan ground to work in him. The one who is experienced in the Lord is able to detect and decipher this peculiar condition. You should learn to use your spirit to touch this unspeakable condition.

Now in fellowshipping with brothers and sisters, if you as God's worker are able to recognize these seven kinds of condition in their spirit, you can apprehend almost all their problems. This I would say especially in reference to the experienced ones among us.

How to Judge with the Spirit

I would now raise a fundamental question for our consideration together. How do you use your spirit to touch another's spirit? How do you judge with your spirit? Let me say at the very outset that for anyone to be able to judge with his spirit, his outward man must be broken. There is no shortcut. He must be dealt with by God, learn all his lessons, and have his outward man broken. Then his spirit can naturally be used. Without the breaking of the outward man his spirit is unusable. The reason why his spirit is unusable is because it is affected by outside influence. His outward man is so strong that his spirit cannot freely launch out. His spirit is bound either by thought or emotion or volition. The outward man is so strong that the spirit of God's children is laid under siege. Therefore, our outward self must be broken. Only after the outward shell is cracked open can the spirit be released. Between you and the other party there is the outward man. In order to touch the other's spirit with your spirit, that outward man of yours has to be broken. Then are you able to know the other's spirit. Without the release of our spirit we lack the basic instrument by which to know others. *

Let us understand that there is an affinity between spirit and spirit. But the outward man is blocking the way. With the breaking of the outward man, though, your spirit can have a greater nearness to God and can have close contact with the spirit of others. It then becomes reasonably easy for your spirit to go forth and help those others. Only those whose outward man is broken can learn to judge with their spirit the feeling and condition of others.

As you listen to people, the first thing to be done is to exercise the spirit. When you are fellowshipping with brothers and sisters and listening to them, you must bring your whole being to a restful calm (this is not passivity). It can be likened to reining in tens of thousands of horses, so as to be able to hearken quietly to people's words. You do not first of all use your mind; you instead use your spirit. For thought is but an auxiliary instrument. If the condition of your spirit is clean, tender and gentle, whatever people say will just naturally touch your spirit. The spirit of the other person will leave an impression on your spirit, causing you to feel either defiled or clean, either resistant or able to be entreated. Your spirit may touch his subjectivity, his emotion or his thought. Your spirit must therefore be altogether quiet, gentle, and clean in order to touch his spirit. Do not use your mind to think; rather, use the

---

* The author has devoted an entire volume to this very important lesson of the Christian life. Please consult Watchman Nee, The Release of the Spirit (Christian Fellowship Publishers, 2000), translated from the Chinese.— Translator

spirit to touch. Such kind of knowing is far more dependable than listening with your mind to a two-hour report by a brother. Knowing by the spirit is the spiritual way.

In this kind of spiritual work we all need to learn humbly and slowly. I do not expect any of us to graduate in a short period. It will require at least three to five years for us to learn. But let us realize and never forget that our thought is not the primary factor here. We cannot put our trust in man's mind for this kind of service. We will go far off the mark if we engage our mind as the primary instrument. And let us never forget, too, that learning to use our spirit in this way is not for our knowledge nor is it for enabling us to pick at people's faults or to criticize them. No, no, no! Such learning is only for the purpose of building up, of helping, and of service. It must in no way be used for tearing down, or for finding out people's faults. To the contrary, in coming to know how to use the spirit to touch the spirit of others, we can render much help to them.

3. Spiritual Judgment:
the Basis of Diagnosis and Judgment

We have already discussed the principles of judgment, the way to discern people's various conditions, and how to use the spirit to touch others in need. We have also pointed out the absolute necessity of our being dealt with before God. Today we intend to inquire into two more things.

Diagnosis

Upon using your spirit to sense another's condition, whether that be in his mind or in his spirit, it does not mean you are now able to diagnose and even heal. Touching man's spirit is one thing; diagnosing is another. Touching man's spirit only gives you the knowledge about the condition of his spirit. How will you interpret his condition as to whether his spirit is right or wrong? How will you know? After you have touched a person's mind and even the spirit behind the mind, how will you diagnose? This is not so easy. You need to have sufficient, comprehensive learning before you can diagnose his sickness. For instance, as you listen to a brother you sense he is one who can quickly lose his temper. But without sufficient experience and learning, you will not be able to tell where the cause of his losing of temper lies. Those who are experienced know that man's temper comes from pride. A quick-tempered man cannot stand any disobedience to his words; he cannot tolerate an unkind word. He looks down upon others. There you touch his pride. It is because there is pride within that he loses his temper. The inexperienced in such matters will not know that loss of temper is but a symptom, not the cause, of a spiritual disease. If a person realizes that loss of temper is but a symptom, he will then try to find its cause in order to heal. But if he does not have sufficient learning, he will fail to pinpoint the cause.

Touching people's spirit with the spirit can be likened to the use of a thermometer in measuring body temperature to determine if any fever is present. Yet you will still need to discover the cause of the fever, since it is but a symptom. The same will be true with the loss of temper. The failure to get to the root cause of bad temper renders healing impossible. What is the use of advising an ill-tempered person to be more patient? Such will be useless for he will simply lose his temper again. If you are ever to know the cause of quick temper in another person, you must learn to know the cause of your own loss of temper. If you are knowledgeable as to your own condition, you will begin to understand that other people are not that much different from you. If you have been able to learn from both yourself and other people, you come to recognize that pride is the cause of bad temper. You may also have discovered that subjectivity, too, may cause the loss of temper: a person may explode if his opinion is not accepted; or if his expectation is not reached, he likewise loses control over his temper.

Brother T. Austin-Sparks once said, "Be observant." We need to learn to observe. In assisting people we must find out the cause of their spiritual sickness before we can help them to go to God and be dealt with. We need to be able to explain both the symptoms and the cause of sickness. Whenever we are faced with a particular issue in brothers and sisters, we should pray to God and examine these brethren. Take crying, for example. You may meet one sister who cries quite easily but another sister who never cries. Your spirit may have already sensed the difference, but what can you do if you fail to judge the cause? You must know by learning that to cry or not to cry is but a symptom. You need to ferret out the cause. Which is correct: to cry or not to cry? Will you encourage people to cry or not to cry? This person's crying is wrong, so you exhort him not to cry. But that other person is wrong in not crying, so you should admonish him to cry. The giving of such counsel has come about because you have come to know by experience where the cause of crying or not crying lies. You have learned this knowledge by first looking at yourself.

Oftentimes you yourself are the best teacher, for you can ask yourself, When did I cry and why? The answer to your inquiry as to why, simply put, came down to the fact that there are two reasons for crying: the first is a crying due to self-love; the second is due to having been dealt with and stricken by God. As to the first reason, a person loves himself so much that he pities himself and cannot deny himself. Such a one will think of himself as too good to incur such trouble as has come his way. The more he muses, the more bitterly he cries. He cannot see himself suffer. And hence, his current trouble stirs up his self-love. And so he cries. Man's self-love often lies in a state of slumber until it is awakened by whatever trouble befalls him. We see, then, how self-love is the first reason. The second reason for crying is as the result of being overthrown by God. At the outset a particular person was not easy to change, he having been hard and unconcerned. He could not be shaken, he not being prone to cry or to laugh. Now having been stricken by God through repeated circumstances of His allowance, the person finds himself unable to overcome God; therefore, he cries.

There are, then, at least these two reasons for crying. If later you see someone crying, you can check his cry against these two reasons in determining why he cried. Crying is not necessarily right, but one who has been stricken by God definitely will cry. Though crying may not always be good, even so, a person who has never cried evidences the fact that he has never been overthrown by God. If someone boasts that he has never cried, that one is undoubtedly a very hard person.

Incredibly, one who is very stubborn before God may pass through many trials and be stricken many times by God and still remain ignorant of any spiritual knowledge as to why all this has been happening. Another person, on the other hand, seems to be soft, and he, too, may go through trials and learn nothing. Normally speaking, many trials and many disciplines of the Holy Spirit should result in many learnings. Yet these people have not learned anything. Why is it that these two persons—one hard in nature and the other one soft—have undergone similar happenings resulting in both having failed to learn any spiritual lesson? We need to find out the cause. We must know not only their symptoms but their causes as well.

Let us review the cases of these two people again. On the one hand, here we have a person who is stubborn and hard before God and reaps no spiritual fruit when under trials. His trials bring in no spiritual blessing from lessons having been learned, only painful experiences. He quarrels with God, is dissatisfied with God's dealing, and disobeys His discipline. He steadfastly believes it is wrong for people to ride above his head; instead, he wants God to make it possible for him to ride over other people's heads. Furthermore, while still under discipline, he lets off steam: he feels misunderstood and considers God to be wrong and he himself to be right. Such a person will never submit himself under God's discipline. He learns absolutely nothing about the place of thanksgiving and praise. Due to the hardness of heart, he learns nothing. On the other hand, here we have another person who, just the opposite, is unusually soft. He too has undergone many trials, having experienced the discipline of the Holy Spirit; and yet he also has garnered for himself no spiritual learning and no spiritual knowledge from his painful experience. The discipline of the Holy Spirit is ineffective in his life as well. Why is this so? In his case it is because he lacks the supply of the ministry of God's word.

In view of all that has been said, therefore, you and I must learn to know people's various conditions and know their meanings. Just knowing that a person has a fever of 100 degrees is not sufficient. You should know its cause. You cannot simply say his fever is due to his physical weakness. You need, on the one side, to observe as does a physician, but on the other side, to have personal dealings before God. After three or five years of diligent observation and lesson-learning discipline, you may be able to diagnose correctly. You yourself must be a gentle and open person before God, acknowledging frequently your proneness to error and your undependableness. With such intensive learning on your own personal level, you can then more readily sense in your spirit the symptom and cause of your brother's weakness and in addition show him the way of healing. In sum, then, in this matter of judging and discerning, the first step is to touch with the spirit; the second is to differentiate with the spirit; the third, to diagnose and find out the cause of sickness; and finally, to heal (for more on the healing step, see the next chapter).

The Foundation of Judgment: Brotherly Love

In learning to recognize people's problems and diagnose their situation, we must realize and continually affirm what is the fundamental basis to all our judging and discerning endeavors. Let us never forget that we do not desire to know and to discern for the sake of seeking or accumulating knowledge about others for ourselves. An abnormal Christian would like to know another's business. But a normal Christian does not seek to know another's condition just for the sake of knowing. Although we indeed must know the conditions of our brethren, it is not out of curiosity or for self-interest. In order to serve and help people, we are compelled to know them. Otherwise, we would rather not know their conditions if such were not necessary. We are busy enough with our own affairs; we have no time to be busybodies. One who desires to know the conditions of others and is continually inquisitive is seriously sick. In fact, he himself needs to be healed! The only reason for knowing is for service and help. I need to know the condition of the brother whom the Lord has placed in my care so that I may help him. Except the Holy Spirit arranges the contact, I have no pleasure in knowing his affairs.

131

To those who are God's workers let me say again and again that I hope you will never have the lust of knowing others' business. I do not want or expect anyone to carelessly gather materials for gossip. Let none of us casually take up the burden of others. May we have no other intention than to help others with whatever knowledge we have gleaned about them.

The social intercourse among the children of God must be based on "love" and not "knowledge." We must never fellowship with brothers and sisters according to knowledge, only according to love. For the basis of Christian fellowship is always to be the latter, never the former. In the world, social intercourse is carried on for the sake of finding bosom friends. But our fellowship is conducted on the basis of brotherly love: we love one another. It is difficult to be true Christians, however, if we base our fellowship on knowledge. If God has not maintained His fellowship with you on the basis of His knowledge of you, then by the same token He will not entrust the knowledge of your brothers and sisters to you if your fellowship with them is based on knowledge. For if it be on that basis, then the more you come to know them the less you will be able to be a Christian: for if it be according to your knowledge of the brethren, you will shake your head at everyone and declare all of them undone. You will shake your head at this brother and that sister till you become so disillusioned that you will hardly be able or even willing to fellowship with any Christian. In the end you will totally shake yourself out. Hence our fellowship with brothers and sisters can only be maintained on the ground of love.

As we have said, then, one's knowledge of a brother is solely for the sake of helping and serving him. You come to know his condition as you work with him. You must never mix up the "knowledge" of the brother with "love" for the brother. God's trusted servants are those who are able to separate "knowledge" and "love" in dealing with people. Those who are unable to separate these two are not fit to be God's servants.

3. Spiritual Judgment:
the Basis of Diagnosis and Judgment

May I warn you beforehand that you are responsible if you wrongly mix up these two. For example, in dealing with your son these two elements of love and knowledge are bound to be present: a father needs to know his son's weaknesses, yet no true father fails to love his son once knowing of his son's weaknesses. The interrelation between father and son is based on love. And love is blind, or should be in this situation. The father's knowledge of his son does not affect his love for his son. And if this be true between father and son, then how can you love your brethren any less than you would in loving your son? What really is fellowshipping in the church on the basis of love? It is simply this, that as you fellowship with your brother, it is done as though you know nothing at all of his weakness or his fault: your fellowship with him is based not on knowledge but on love. And that must always be the basis of our fellowship together.

Judging according to knowledge will make of us politicians, which is not Christian. A person who reaches the age of around fifty is experienced and wise. He is one who will not be easily deceived or fooled in the latter part of his life. Now the world would call such a person a clever old man; for such cleverness is the way of the world. However, no Christian— though he knows so much and so well about others—may follow this clever worldly pathway. Today our knowledge of brothers and sisters may be meager, but after several years of dealing with brethren our knowledge of them will greatly increase. By that time, we will be able to know a person after only a few words of conversation. And the consequent danger is that it will become increasingly difficult for us to love that person. Let not such a thing happen in our midst. If we Christians treat brothers and sisters according to knowledge, it is true we may avoid many crosses and incur far less trouble than were we to follow the way of love; nevertheless, if we treat our brother according to knowledge, we too will become clever—and even tricky—old hands. That is not progression, it is regression.

We must ever keep ourselves in the love of God. Whatever knowledge the Lord gives us about brothers and sisters is for the sake of healing ministry. I do not need to remind you that once a worldling is betrayed, he finds it extremely difficult, if not impossible, to love anymore. He becomes fearful. This is not to be so, however, with a Christian; for among believers in Christ love must reign supreme, no matter what. Let us not become clever because we have the opportunity to know brothers and sisters so well. If our knowledge of them is only obtained for the purpose of protecting ourselves from being cheated by them, or less bothered by them, then our knowledge merely helps us to be a clever person who can thereby avoid unwanted problems.

Let us ask God to grant us greater love for the brethren. We should pray that our love for them may surpass our knowledge of them. May our love of the brethren transcend all. Let us also pray that our love for them will not be affected by any cleverness we might be tempted to indulge in so as to make life easier for ourselves. To know others is to facilitate our service to them, not to lessen our trouble. Let us ask God to so fill our hearts with love for others in the body of Christ that we seem to be totally ignorant of their weaknesses, faults and problems. If such an attitude be taken, then this is truly otherworldly in character. Let us bear in mind that the more we know our brethren the narrower will be our way: we must never be afraid of being bothered or cheated or defrauded or even betrayed: instead, let our love overcome all. In the end, "brotherly love" is the only way.

4. Spiritual Judgment: Healing

The Way to Healing

After you have used the spirit to touch the conditions and problems of the brothers and sisters, you may begin to diagnose and show them the way to healing. This is easy to say, but in real situations it is rather hard to convince people. In order to help them towards deliverance, you yourself must have sufficient experience that can enable you to speak so clearly and thoroughly that it gives light to them to be delivered. The difficulties in helping people are: one, our insufficient experience; and two, our inadequate words. If our experience and words are ample enough, we shall be able to cause people to see light.

I recall many years ago when in Shanghai that I had no way to help a certain brother. This was due to my insufficient experience. His will was extremely strong and he was proud and quick-tempered. Some people are quick-tempered, but they are not proud. This brother was strong-willed and quick-tempered. So he was not easy to deal with. For a person whose will is strong, yet whose emotion is not easily stirred, his problem remains in himself. If a person like this loses his temper, a simple confession will usually come forth and the problem is resolved. But a strong-willed and quick-tempered person is also very subjective. When he is aroused, he maintains that his temper is justified. Therefore, he will not repent. Such a combination creates a major problem.

Some persons may have only one problem, others may have two or three problems, which can impinge on one another to aggravate their difficulties. In medicine, sometimes a combination of diseases makes a deteriorating physical condition difficult to cure, because each disease affects the other and heightens the overall sickness. Yet this is also true in human nature. You need to understand the interaction of different characteristics. A strong-willed, proud and quick-tempered individual needs very intensive handling.

Now after you have apprehended a brother's condition, you have two alternative ways by which to help.

1. Admonish

The first way to help is by admonition. You show the brother the way of deliverance. This one has never seen light, so he is ignorant of himself and no one has ever spoken frankly to him. As you talk with him, you will present before him what you have seen. You will tell him your own experience. You advise him to allow himself to be dealt with by God, to accept the discipline of the Holy Spirit. For his way is not straight: he lives by his mind and emotion, his spirit is weak, he has flaws before God, and he has refused the Spirit's discipline on many occasions. If your light is sufficiently accurate, you can rescue him. But you yourself must not be confused. Light always brings in deliverance. Light also brings in release. You can invite him to come and have pointed out to him those things about which he has rejected the discipline of the Spirit. Your words of admonition need to be positive. They must not be casual, but be always exact. You prove your words by citing several instances wherein he has refused the discipline of the Holy Spirit. Few make errors by chance; instead, most commit temperamental errors. The slow are always slow, and the quick are always quick. Temperamental error is a human problem. So, you offer help to rectify his temperamental error, not his occasional fault.

Now in our giving help, it cannot be general but needs to be specific and with definite procedure. *Number one*, take down the facts. You should prepare a notebook to record the facts. For example, let us say that a brother speaks inaccurately or tells lies. The first time you heard him do so you wrote down what he said and where he said it. For if this is a flaw in character, he will again say inaccurate words or speak falsehoods. You record his inaccurate or lying words time and again, perhaps up to ten or twenty times. By this account you will know that this is his character flaw. And then, as opportunity presents itself, at the right time you will be able to show him how inaccurate or false have been his words.

Number two, you yourself must be strengthened within. You need to be built up before God before you have the strength to help others. As the records in your notebook mount up, your inner strength needs to be increased. You must climb higher and higher, your strength becoming stronger and stronger till your inner fortitude is sufficient enough to deal with him and render help.

Number three, wait for an appropriate time to talk with him. In the meantime, while waiting, your inner burden can keep increasing. You ask God to arrange an opportunity to speak with him. Then, as you talk with him, pay attention to the following points: (1) Say to him, "I wish to speak a few words with you. You need not even answer. Yet whether what I say to you is right or wrong, you need to go before God to consider what I have said." Do not give ground to him to argue. (2) Say also to him, "All these words are spoken for your benefit. I have no interest in meddling in your business. I do not thoughtlessly interfere with another's affairs. It is solely for the sake of helping you." (3) You may also add, "I say these words without there being any personal motive involved." Recall to him the mounting incidents of his lying or speaking inaccurately. And cause him to see that he is an inveterate liar. Say to him, "You need to repent before God, otherwise you have no way through." During your conversation, you should not stop short of dealing strongly with his lying and/or inaccurate speech. Yet concerning any other faults, you need only to mention them. Serious sin must be vigorously denounced, whereas much lighter sin needs only a slight reprimand.

2. Reprove

The people with problems whom we encounter may be generally divided into three groups. The first group is composed of people with little problems. All you need to do is to approach him personally and point out his small problem. You can deal with the situation alone. The second group consists of people with a major problem—a problem which has become deeply rooted in their life. You will need to use weighty words to bring such ones back. And if it subsequently becomes clear to you that you by yourself are inadequate, you should invite two or three brothers with experience to go with you and speak these weighty words in their presence. And finally, the third group is comprised of people whose problems are so deep that they cannot be easily changed. In that case, you need to bring with you two or three other brothers for talking with such a one. There has arisen such repulsion in you against this particular problem that you are well-nigh ready to reprove him with severity. You have the judgment within you, and you also have the word of reproof. In the presence of these other brothers you not only admonish him, you strictly reprove him. For as you speak to him you are representing God in reproving him. In reproving, you need to have the wrath of God in you. If he listens to you, he shall be delivered from his problem.

How can a person overcome weakness? How can his problem be solved? His weakness and his problem are resolved under an awesome light. When God's light comes, it provides man with no place to hide. All that is not of God is dried up and withered. And the stronger the light, the quicker the withering. Whether or not a brother's difficulty is solved depends on the degree of light we give. Leprosy in its hidden stage cannot be healed; but once it is fully exposed, the leprosy is healed. In order to give sufficiently strong light, we ourselves must not harbor any personal feeling or have any personal interest. We need to be purely for the brother's sake. If any personal feeling or personal interest is present, you and I are unable to solve people's problems. By speaking frankly to our brethren and bringing their weakness into God's light, we can deliver them from their problem that can now be withered beyond revival.

Some may ask why it is necessary to bring along two or three other brothers? When one person speaks alone, sometimes the light does not appear to be strong enough. The bringing of two or three others into the picture is to increase the measure of light, to heighten the problem present in the opposite party, to amplify the exposure of that difficulty, and to aggravate his shame. Thus will he be broken at once, and be delivered from his problem. The light brought in by two or three others is stronger than the light of just one person. The issue now is whether that person will accept the dealing.

It is also asked, Why is there the need of reproof? In the Bible there are many incidents recorded wherein reproving words were required. Today in the Church, there are few of us, if any, who dare to reprimand people. And why? Because our own life is not right, and so we are not found worthy to dispense reproof. For as soon as we would reprove others, we would in reality be reproving our own selves. Moreover, we have our personal feeling, and therefore we cannot reprove others. To reprove others we must not bring any personal feeling into the matter at hand. The reproofs in the Bible do not involve personal feeling. They are all for God, for the Church, and for the brothers and sisters.

For the benefit of your brethren, you cannot but speak frankly. To reprimand others, you must deeply hate the particular matter at issue. You must have such strong revulsion against the error that you are very angry at it. Unless you yourself are such before God, you have no way to scold others. If your words come from God, then as you speak severely to the troubled one in the presence of other brothers, light will shine upon that one and blind him. And after two or three days, he will gradually see light. Something has been cut away from him: a wound has been inflicted upon him: and his problem has withered away.

You will notice that I entitled these messages under the general rubric of "spiritual judgment." And one of the various aspects in God's judgment is His wrath. As He judges, all is cleansed. One day when God's anger is totally provoked, this entire world will be purified and Satan's work will vanish from the scene forever. It is a good thing if after following the Lord for thirty or fifty years, a person may be called upon to represent God's wrath. The (righteous) anger of elderly brothers can deliver some brethren from their problems. But younger brothers should not be tempted in this respect. Your time to represent God's wrath has not yet come. You who are younger should instead learn to bear the cross and accept the discipline of the Holy Spirit. This is because currently you can only exhibit anger that comes from yourself, and thus you will find it necessary to go before God to confess. But with some elderly brothers, they may indeed exhibit anger, but because it is from God they do not need to return to Him to confess. For anger which comes from God is vastly different from anger which comes from self. Whatever anger or loss of temper which comes from self needs to be confessed; otherwise, one cannot have fellowship with God. But whatever wrath comes from God need not be repented of, and one's communion with Him remains unbroken. Ordinary brethren can only admonish, they cannot reprove the brother who needs help. Those elderly among us who have godly confidence within may alone judge with the wrath of God the difficulties of the brethren.

I very rarely mention these matters because they are not common. We must always exercise judgment with fear and trembling. We should have more learning at the hands of Almighty God.

Prayer:

O Lord, I pray especially for the brothers and sisters gathered here, that they may be delivered inwardly. I pray that they may be able, without self-love or despair, to know themselves before the Lord so thoroughly that they can help many by bringing them to the way of light and out of the way of darkness. May they live day by day in You, and not in themselves. Cause them, Lord, to receive greater enlightenment in You, to enter more into the discipline of the Holy Spirit, and learn to fear You and be delivered from self as they seek to serve You and the body of Christ. Amen.

TITLES AVAILABLE
from Christian Fellowship Publishers

By Watchman Nee

Aids to "Revelation"
Amazing Grace
Back to the Cross
A Balanced Christian Life
The Better Covenant
The Body of Christ: A Reality
The Character of God's Workman
Christ the Sum of All Spiritual Things
The Church and the Work – 3 Vols
The Church in the Eternal Purpose of God
"Come, Lord Jesus"
The Communion of the Holy Spirit
The Finest of the Wheat – Vol. 1
The Finest of the Wheat – Vol. 2
From Faith to Faith
From Glory to Glory
Full of Grace and Truth – Vol. 1
Full of Grace and Truth – Vol. 2
Gleanings in the Fields of Boaz
The Glory of His Life
God's Plan and the Overcomers
God's Work
Gospel Dialogue
Grace Abounding
Grace for Grace
Heart-to-Heart Talks
Interpreting Matthew
Journeying towards the Spiritual
The King and the Kingdom of Heaven
The Latent Power of the Soul
Let Us Pray

The Life That Wins
The Lord My Portion
The Messenger of the Cross
The Ministry of God's Word
My Spiritual Journey
The Mystery of Creation
Powerful According to God
Practical Issues of This Life
The Prayer Ministry of the Church
The Release of the Spirit
Revive Thy Work
The Salvation of the Soul
The Secret of Christian Living
Serve in Spirit
The Spirit of Judgment
The Spirit of the Gospel
The Spirit of Wisdom and Revelation
Spiritual Authority
Spiritual Discernment
Spiritual Exercise
Spiritual Knowledge
The Spiritual Man
Spiritual Reality or Obsession
Take Heed
The Testimony of God
The Universal Priesthood of Believers
Whom Shall I Send?
The Word of the Cross
Worship God
Ye Search the Scriptures

The Basic Lesson Series
Vol. 1 - A Living Sacrifice
Vol. 2 - The Good Confession
Vol. 3 - Assembling Together
Vol. 4 - Not I, But Christ
Vol. 5 - Do All to the Glory of God
Vol. 6 - Love One Another

ORDER FROM: 11515 Allecingie Parkway Richmond, VA 23235
www.c-f-p.com – 804-794-5333

TITLES AVAILABLE
from Christian Fellowship Publishers

By Stephen Kaung

"But We See Jesus"—*the Life of the Lord Jesus*
Discipled to Christ—*As Seen in the Life of Simon Peter*
God's Purpose for the Family
The Gymnasium of Christ
In the Footsteps of Christ
The Key to "Revelation" – Vol. 1
The Key to "Revelation" – Vol. 2
Men After God's Own Heart—*Eight Biographies from the Book of Genesis*
New Covenant Living & Ministry
Now We See the Church—*the Life of the Church, the Body of Christ*
Shepherding
The Songs of Degrees—*Meditations on Fifteen Psalms*
The Splendor of His Ways—*Seeing the Lord's End in Job*

The "God Has Spoken" Series
Seeing Christ in the Old Testament, Part One
Seeing Christ in the Old Testament, Part Two
Seeing Christ in the New Testament

ORDER FROM: 11515 Allecingie Parkway Richmond, VA 23235
www.c-f-p.com – 804-794-5333